It Has Nothing To Do With Age

By Frank Lieberman, PhD

WinterGoose
Publishing

Winter Goose Publishing
2701 Del Paso Road, 130-92
Sacramento, CA 95835

www.wintergoosepublishing.com
Contact Information: info@wintergoosepublishing.com

It Has Nothing To Do With Age
COPYRIGHT © 2011 by Frank Lieberman

First Edition, September, 2011
Cover Art by Winter Goose Publishing

Typeset by Victoriakumar Yallamelli for
Winter Goose Publishing

Published in the United States of America
ISBN: 978-0-9836764-0-9

Dedication

To the memory of my mother.

Table of Contents

Foreword

I met Frank in 2002 when making my documentary Running Madness. This is a film about the elite and often bizarre world of ultra running, and Frank was one of the competitors. I was immediately drawn to his story and his sense of humor. I felt he had real insight into the mind of an extreme athlete which was both experiential and academic; a potent combination. When Frank shared with me that he had written a book, I was eager to read it and I am thrilled to say it lives up to my impression of him. Frank is a man who seeks truth and works to heal himself and those around him. In this gem of a book, he posits that as we age we don't lose our capacity to grow and change and realize our dreams; that it's only our mind that can limit our potential. Frank's own story and those he's collected, beautifully illustrate the peaks and valleys we all face, as well as the inevitable stumbles. Each page is a celebration of the triumph of the human spirit. Perhaps for many of us it's not an ultra marathon, but we can all learn from these stories and find our own trail. Frank's story will inspire and provide hope for living through life's changes with grace, humor and humility.

Susan Cohn Rockefeller

I

What Makes Frank Run?

Frank Lieberman is mentally and physically strong, tough, athletic, health-conscious and competitive. He is goal-oriented, persevering, determined, and passionate, while defying his age. Born on November 26, 1939 in Detroit, Michigan, this PhD psychologist is about 5-feet 9-inces tall and weighs approximately 165 pounds.

I'm Frank Lieberman, and these pages contain the profile of my life as a senior ultra athlete. My purpose here is not only to entertain and educate you about my path and the journey of other ultra athletes, but to also give you inspiration and guidance in your own life. Your goal may not be ultra sports, but perhaps just making that one step toward a healthier, more joyful life.

In the year 2000, at the age of 60, I completed the Tevis Cup, a 100-mile endurance horse event over the Sierra Nevada Mountains. This is a grueling challenge that must be accomplished within 24 hours to qualify for completion. At the age of 62, I was a division winner in the 100-mile Western States Endurance Run, the ultra marathon known as the toughest on the planet. These two events have attracted a remarkable range of competitors from all over the globe, and I am one of about 45 individuals in the world to have earned belt buckles in both the Tevis Cup and the Western States 100-mile Endurance Run.

At the age of 68, I came in first place in the Swanton Pacific 100-mile Ride & Tie, along with team members Jonathan Jordan and my Arabian mare "Gypsy." A Ride & Tie is three athletes-two people and one horse-competing over a designated distance; one person runs and the other rides, and then they trade off during the competitive race.

With those three accomplishments, I became one of only four individuals in the world to have completed the Tevis Cup, the 100-mile

Western States Endurance Run, and the Swanton Pacific 100-mile Ride & Tie. Proudly, I'm the only individual in their 60s to have ever completed these three events.

If you were an equestrian, you would more than likely know about the Tevis Cup. If you were an ultra endurance runner, you would be familiar with the Western States Run. If you knew about both endurance riding and ultra running, you might be knowledgeable about Ride & Tie. Similarities in each of these events are as follows: all take place on mountain trails and are 100 miles in distance; each event has about a 50% completion rate; all three were created within the last 60 years; and they are known as the grandfathers of their sport. Each of these events has competitor entry criteria, each has a completion time cut-off, and each is to be completed within one day. Both Ride & Tie and the Tevis Cup have a 24-hour time limit while the Western States Endurance Run has a 30-hour cut-off.

It's likely that most people do not know about these three extreme amateur sports or the other unique sport activities found in this book. As you read these chapters, you will discover what drives the men and women who compete in these difficult sports as well as the Dipsea and the Hawaiian Ironman, details about the sports themselves, and about the history of the competitions. The water sports of outrigger canoe paddling, rowing, and sculling round out the list of extreme competitions.

I believe the individuals in this book, all ranging in age from 65 to 85, are interesting, inspiring, compassionate, driven, and disciplined people. Yes, they have accomplished incredible feats in their senior years, but they are also mortals faced with typical challenges we all confront in life—financial woes, family issues, divorce, health problems, and even death. As life deals out these cards, sometimes it's those challenges that cause people to push themselves, ultimately escalating to ultra sports.

As I've experienced from writing this book, I hope that you'll also identify and draw strength from these inspirational stories. I encourage you to use the information to your advantage and let these role models assist you in establishing a roadmap for developing meaning and passion in your life. It is never too late to begin.

Just because we age does not mean we have to retire or stop living productively. We can also evolve and become an active outdoor participant in meaningful and healthy events. Noted attorney Eugene D'Ablemont, age 70, was forced to retire from his New York law firm even though he was a partner there for four decades, and definitely didn't want to retire. Essentially our society forced him to step down, pushing aside the facts that he was still productive, successful, and engaged in and committed to his profession. Our society views aging in terms of numbers rather than ability. The question remains, who should make the decision? In my opinion, we need to challenge the notion of how this arbitrary, stand-alone number is the basis for retirement.

Is there more to life than work in today's world? Look around and you'll see 'older' individuals being more active, acting younger, and participating in more adventurous activities. Take Hse Telesmanich, for example. At 90 years of age, she sprained her ankle while hiking in South Africa. Was her sprained ankle a problem that got in the way of her hiking? No! She said, "I got very good at hopping on one foot."

When Tom Lackey was a youthful 89, he stood atop the wing of a biplane while it was flying across the English Channel. Why did he do it? His explanation was that he took up wing-walking as a way to deal with the grief of losing his wife. There are, of course, simpler and less dangerous ways to deal with loss. You might become like Jon Mendes, age 90, who entered the New York City Marathon in 2010, or even like Canadian Olga Kotelko, age 91, who still competes and holds the record for the javelin throw, 100 meter dash, shot put, and the high jump in Masters track competition for her age group. At the moment, she is the age group. Who knows, you might become a competitor in the centenarian age group too.

Even Hollywood depicts rugged action stars in retirement age as adventurous and principled. To illustrate, the 1992 movie "Unforgiven" was directed by and starred Clint Eastwood. In this film, Clint, as William Munny, was a retired gunman. He did not stay retired, and after a few attempts, he was able to get back on his horse to gallop away and hand out frontier justice when it was necessary. "High Noon," a movie made in 1952, was about Will Kane, portrayed by Gary Cooper. In this film, Will was about to retire from being the town marshal. However, on his last day on the job, he learned that a man he sent to prison years earlier was returning on the noon train to seek revenge. Did Cooper fight or take flight? He stayed to fight—and won. In 1979, the film "Going in Style" was about three older men trying to subsist, rather unsuccessfully, on Social Security income. They then robbed a bank and brought excitement into their lives. Even Hollywood can tell a good story about people who age without losing relevance, even if they employ aggression and violence in their films, in addition to responsibility, loyalty, and friendship.

Over the years Time Magazine has had a number of interesting commentaries and articles in reference to aging. They reported that only about 30% of aging is genetically based, which means that other variables are under our control. Let me repeat this fact: Some 70% of how we age is under our control! When people truly grasp that significant fact, they'll realize that we are not just a product of our genes, and that we can take an active stance in how our life unfolds. It's up to us to make the best of our lives and our health. If we can change our thinking, we can change our behavior, and in my professional life, that's exactly how I've observed the way transformations unfold: change in thinking results in behavioral change. We have conscious control of our thoughts, which means we can plan, set goals, and make changes in our thinking and therefore our behavior.

One step in achieving a longer lifespan, according to Time, is to "get back some of what we lose by our overfed, overstressed, and underactive lifestyles." Television's popular Dr. Mehmet Oz gave his prescription for living long and living well. He suggests we get daily rigor-

5. Participate in outdoor activities to help nurture spirituality.

6. For a way to escape, read about other people's adventures.

7. Find inspiration and motivation through the illuminating profiles of eight remarkable senior athletes found within this book.

II

Of Triumph and Tragedy

To start my tale, I'm going back to 1980 when I re-married and moved from San Leandro to Fremont; both cities are in the San Francisco Bay Area. I was a psychologist enjoying my private practice.

I took up horseback riding lessons at a nearby stable and I remember that during the first or second lesson my trainer told me I had a good sitting trot. I was pleased, and later I realized that she was generous with her feedback. Unfortunately, I was unable to properly post when my horse was at the trot; posting is a rise-and-sit motion in concert with the strides of the horse.

After four or five lessons I got more and more into it. My wife at the time bought an Arabian horse, and I leased a horse for my lessons. I preferred being on the trail rather than the arena which to me proved to be boring.

One Saturday, my wife, another trainer, and I left the arena for a trail ride. My wife was in the lead and leaned forward when they approached a steep incline. When her horse reached a level plateau, he bucked and she landed headfirst on the rocky ground. She was in excruciating pain and we took her to the emergency room at Washington Hospital where she was put in intensive care. Her injuries included a broken palette, which needed to be wired shut, and a fractured wrist. Needless to say, the horse was sold.

She recovered and went through rehabilitation, but she never lost her dream of riding horses. During our gentle re-entry into the horse world, we heard about a cowboy who had a ranch in Coyote near San Jose, California. An older man, Veryl Lybert was originally from Alberta, Canada. He had this wonderful ranch property that included Quarter Horses, draft horses, chickens, and Border Collie dogs. He hosted parties for corporations where people were entertained by a petting zoo and roping demonstrations, and feasted on terrific BBQs. This cowboy was no nonsense, talked straight, and was right to the point. He knew my wife had experienced a serious horse accident. When we arrived to evaluate and possibly purchase one or two of his horses, she said to him, "I would like to ride Smoke in the arena." Veryl replied, "You've done the arena already." So we saddled up the horses and went on a trail ride accompanied by Veryl and his two Border Collies.

After a couple of months of riding with Veryl—my wife on Smoke, and me on a Quarter Horse named Nowata, we began to really get some trail riding experience. Of course, one of the dogs usually accompanied us on the trail rides. I liked having a Border Collie along on the rides and you can probably guess the breed of my first dog. Yep, a Border Collie; we named her Scampi.

After a while, we learned to ride the trails without Veryl. One humorous episode was when we stopped for a picnic, our first with the horses, and instead of tying the horses to a tree, we put hobbles on their front feet. Hobbles are a one-piece device with a loop for each front foot, which means (in theory) they can't travel far or fast. Still being a city slicker, I'm not sure what I did wrong, but the horses took off. I was amazed to see front feet moving so fast in unison as they left us in the dust. We eventually caught up to the grazing horses and learned a valuable lesson: tie your horse. I must have seen too many western movies where the horses stayed near the rider, seemingly untied, and apparently I thought that would just magically happen.

Veryl invited us to assist the other nearby ranchers in rounding up the cows that required branding and vaccinations. I thought, wow! That would be fun—chasing cows just like a real cowboy. We were real city slickers and thought it would be easy! But being a cowboy is harder than you think, believe me.

Eventually it became time to cut the umbilical cord with Veryl, purchase the horses and find a stable for them. We were excited to purchase Smoke and Nowata from him.

Veryl delivered Smoke and Nowata to a nearby boarding stable close to Fremont. Eventually we had to buy our own horse trailer and truck.

Mind you, my experience at this point was limited trail riding and I didn't know how to load a horse into a trailer. Picture this: a brand-new Logan walk-in horse trailer, two horses, and two greenhorns. Somehow or other, Smoke managed to load himself by simply walking into the trailer. However, I could not get Nowata into the trailer, he just wouldn't go. If you've ever experienced a horse that did not want to get into a trailer, you know what I mean. The expression "you can lead a horse to water but you can't make him drink" fits here. I found the owner of a nearby stable, a John Wayne type, and asked him for help. What a mistake that turned out to be. He and some other people attempted to muscle my horse into the trailer while Nowata resisted beyond measure. They put the lead rope into his mouth while pulling him forward and pushing him from behind. The horse was mostly in the trailer but was thrashing and pulling back even though he was tied to a ring in the trailer. The butt chain was put across and attached to the back end of the trailer. Nowata simply dropped his hind end and in doing so wedged it underneath the butt chain and was now stuck. In moving backward he seemed to lose his balance and fell out of the trailer and onto the ground. He could not stand, and he repeatedly thrashed about, hitting his head on the ground over and over. Later, I was told he had severed his spinal cord. I was in shock, horrified and questioning what to do. I was paralyzed and felt helpless. Somebody called a veterinarian, who arrived and immediately injected Nowata to euthanize him. My first horse, my first loading experience, and it turned out to be a nightmare. I still have horrifying memories of that event. Even now, I worry about loading any horse into a trailer and get very nervous and uncomfortable. The memory of what Nowata went through and my experience of being helpless was a nightmare that stays with me today. My poor horse's death could have been prevented. Shortly after my horse's death, a friend gave me her Quarter Horse gelding named Leo. He was a terrific horse who taught me a lot on the trail. He was well-schooled and excellent on trail rides. I rode him for many miles in the Bay Area hills and around the nearby grounds of the stable. I became more and more competent as an equestrian.

While at the stable, a friend told us about the North American Trail Ride Conference (NATRC) competitions. In this sport, the horse and rider are judged on how well they perform point-to-point on a designated trail. The horse is judged by a veterinarian on physical parameters (pulse, respiration, soundness, etc.) as well as behavior, and the rider is critiqued by a lay judge on criteria such as trail etiquette, stabling, equitation, etc. The judges are typically hidden from view; you couldn't see them but they could see you. There was a minimum and a maximum time for the distance; if you rode too fast or too slow you were disqualified. You had to assess your speed and time over the trail, among other strategic plans. Those who did well would get brightly colored ribbons as awards. I did not like being judged nor did I like getting a report card, so I rebelled. One time a judge remarked, "Frank, wear your number so we can see it!"

After a few years I was content with trail riding and also competed in two limited distance endurance events of 25 miles on my Quarter Horse. I also purchased new motorcycles year after year. My unrest was clear but I was not dealing with the source. My happiness with my marriage did not change because I purchased a new motorcycle, or went on countless vacations to Mexico, Hawaii, or various ports of call.

At first it was enjoyable riding horses with my wife, but even that became unpleasant. All the signs were there of a marriage on the rocks and dissolving. Working long hours in my psychotherapy practice also didn't solve any problems. I was troubled but was still not willing to get a divorce at that time.

I entered a 25-mile limited-distance endurance ride in early 1997 called the Mustang Classic at Mount Hamilton in San Jose, California. This endurance ride hosted a Ride & Tie event at the same time as the endurance ride. I had heard about Ride & Tie and was under the impression that it was an event only for elite athletes. I thought that anyone who participated in this event was likely to be lean, tall and a superior runner. Foolish me, I did not think about the necessary equestrian skills that would be needed as well. At this time I was not running nor in great physical condition. I think subconsciously I was entertaining the idea of competing in a Ride & Tie and that those thoughts were just waiting to erupt to the surface.

I completed the 25-mile limited distance endurance ride and waited for the awards dinner that followed. Camped next to me were two lean, bearded men, Tony Brickel and Jeff Windenhausen. As it turned out, Tony was younger than me and Jeff a little older. These two men had completed the Ride & Tie and were partners. They were friendly and outgoing, and didn't exactly fit the age-image I had of Ride & Tie people. Tony and Jeff looked older to me, but looks can be deceiving. Not every one of the Ride & Tie types who walked by were thin and athletic looking. There were different body types. I believed that I could spot an elite athlete by their appearance. How naïve I was at the time.

As I engaged Tony and Jeff in conversation, along came Kurt Riffle and Robert Eichstaedt from Ride & Tie. Kurt was the president of the Ride & Tie Association. We talked about Ride & Tie and even though I was not a runner at that time, I was recruited because I had a horse and some interest. I agreed to enter the Quicksilver Ride & Tie in San Jose, and Kurt volunteered to find a partner for me. My task at that point was to start running and training to get in condition for the event held in May. Unfortunately, I was not able to run any of the hills, but I found that I could run the flats, so when I started running and training I simply walked the hills. I didn't know much about training myself, or conditioning at that time, but it all began with trial and error. I don't remember much during that month before my first Ride & Tie; the time went by fast. Kurt said, "Show up and your partner will be there." Okay, I can ride, and all I need to do is to begin running.

Per the Ride & Tie Association, here's what I learned: The objective is to get all three team members (two humans and one horse) across the course by alternating riding and running. One team member starts out running, the other starts on the horse and rides down the marked trail as far as the rider thinks their partner can run at a good pace. At that strategic point the rider stops, safely ties the horse to a tree, and continues down the trail on foot. The team member who started on foot soon finds the horse and unties it, mounts and rides to catch the runner up ahead. On a 'flying tie exchange,' no one stops, but the rider can also ride further and then tie the horse and continue running. This process of 'riding and tying' continues for the entire length of the course until all three members have crossed the finish line.

My limited run training was now complete. I had a partner, and I knew that in Ride & Tie the team starts the race together and finishes the race together. What I didn't know was: how long do I ride before I tie the horse? How many exchanges do the partners make? When should I gallop my horse? Should I tie my horse close to another horse? Under what conditions should I not tie my horse? I began thinking of the Dionne Warwick-Burt Bacharach song, "Do You Know the Way to San Jose?" This is all part of my nervousness. Who was I kidding and who made up this crazy sport?

In 1959 Bud Johns, a freelance writer was researching an area in Southern California near San Diego. In searching for historical information, he found a 1933 newspaper article about an incident that took place in Pine Valley in the late 1800s. The article was about horse rustlers who made off with a herd of horses with the exception of one lone steed. The owner of the stolen herd and his son, along with the one remaining horse, went to retrieve the stolen horses. When the father rode, the son either walked or ran. When the son got on the horse, the father either walked or ran. The good guys eventually tracked down the bad guys and got their horses back. That, my friend, is the first recorded history of Ride & Tie.

Bud, a sports writer in a previous life, thought to himself, "This ride and tie idea could become a race competition." In 1969, Bud was in management with Levi Strauss & Co. with the title 'Communication Director.' One day Bud and his group were brainstorming about how to market and promote the rough-and-tough image of Levi's jeans, and in 1971, Levi's, who sponsored the event for 17 consecutive years, had its first Ride & Tie in St. Helena, California. In that first Levi's Ride & Tie on June 6, 1971, endurance riders Jim

Larimer and Hal Hall came in first place. Sixty-six teams entered that 28-mile race.

On August 27, 1972, the second Levi's Ride & Tie race, this time 29 miles, was held in Alturas, California. A man by the name of Gordon "Gordy" Ainsley and his partner David Roos came in fifth place. You will hear more about Gordy later. In 1973, on June 10th, the third annual Levi's Ride & Tie was held in Angels Camp, California, and was 25 miles in distance. These athletes were pioneers both in Ride & Tie and ultra running. The 40 years of Ride & Tie history depicts many outstanding athletes.

Bud Johns told me the story about an elite athlete and Olympian named Tom Laris. The story goes that Tom had to run 30 some miles during a Ride & Tie without his partner or horse. After successfully crossing the finish line in top position, he looked around and watched other competitors who took three to four hours longer to complete. Amazed at their attitude, this Olympian runner joined these folks back out on the trail, just to experience the sheer joy they had in participating. He remarked, "They are having the time of their lives!" Tom said that he enjoyed being with these cheerful participants, and kindly acknowledged these people who found their own 'personal best' and glory in showing up at the starting line and having fun throughout the event. This sport, Tom now understood, was for both extreme winning athletes and those who cared enough to give it their very best to simply finish.

Bud also told me that he first met my soon to be good friend, veterinarian and competitor Jim Steere after that first Ride & Tie. Jim became Ride & Tie's head veterinarian starting in 1972 and had been Bud's good friend for a long time.

These events create camaraderie among competitors and all the volunteers. The bond created on and off the trail is almost indescribable, and the word 'family' is often mentioned among these athletes and supporters. After decades of being devoted friends, in 2010 Bud Johns was one of the presenters at Jim Steere's memorial, a friend and 'family member' to the end.

III

In the Beginning: My First Ride & Tie

May 1997 came fast. I was extremely anxious, wondering what I had gotten myself into. My self-doubts exploded: Can I do this? Am I ready? Will my partner be there for the race start? Can he ride my horse? Will we be good partners? What about my horse Running Bear, is he ready? What will happen to Running Bear when I tie him to a tree, will he go nuts when other horses race by?

The day came when I arrived at Almaden Park in San Jose, California, for the Quicksilver Ride & Tie race. It was apparent that I was nervous and full of negative thoughts. I parked my Ford Bronco, took Running Bear out of the horse trailer, and began to groom him. My new friend Kurt Riffle came over and introduced me to my partner for the day. "Meet Russ Kiernan," he announced. Russ was tall, thin and athletic looking. He looked the part and was dressed like a runner. He fit my perception of a Ride & Tie athlete; so far so good, I thought. One of the first things he mentioned was for me not to worry about running up the hills because he ran them very well. I was pleased to hear that. This Ride & Tie event was 22 miles, and was even more rugged because of the hills.

The race started with Cardiac Hill. Thank God I began the race in the saddle on Running Bear and I didn't have to deal with that "Hill" on foot. A number of participants were on excited horses with their race partners stretching and warming-up nearby. Rather unceremoniously, a few of the participants yelled to signify the start and off we went! The horses were galloping madly and the runners quickly got out of the way of the charging steeds. It was like a stampede. Heck, it was a stampede! I looked around, held tightly onto the reins, and began galloping Running Bear up Cardiac Hill. What a rush! I was scanning ahead, making sure I was not running into anything or smashing into other horses. I had to maneuver around those horses that had stopped for a hand tie, where the horse is held by a volunteer in anticipation of the arrival of the team's second person on foot. Gratefully, I did not collide with any horses. I am not sure how long I had ridden as it all happened so fast, but then I saw volunteer Robert Eichstaedt on my left, slightly off the trail. Thank goodness he was out of the way of charging horses. I quickly dismounted and handed the reins to Robert to hold for a hand tie. I hoped that my partner Russ wasn't far behind and could easily find Running Bear attached to Robert, mount up and quickly ride on.

A hand tie, I quickly discovered, was allowed only at the beginning of the event. With a hand tie, a person literally takes the place of a tree. The person can also help you mount the excited steed. Believe me that was important, especially at the beginning of the race. Attempting to mount a horse that was racing around in a circle was quite a sight and what you would expect to see among circus clowns clamoring about in the big top. Robert said confidently, "I'll take care of your horse; you continue running and Russ will catch you." I was conscious but not fully cognizant. With all the horses racing by I became anxious; it seemed chaotic to say the least. I started running and I don't remember how far or how long I ran, but I knew that it wasn't for a terribly long time.

Pretty soon Russ, on Running Bear, caught up to me. He rode by and yelled, "I'll tie him up ahead!" I remember feeling tired at that moment, breathing heavily, my legs felt weighted down and I was already exhausted. This sport was not easy, nor for the faint of heart. As I ran up the trail, I saw Running Bear looking back at me, standing calmly with his tie rope wrapped around a tree limb. I mounted, trotted and galloped up the trail, and eventually caught up to Russ. We did an exchange, and I was back on the ground again running.

We made several exchanges before we reached the veterinary checkpoint at approximately the 10-mile mark of the race, where I found my horse. The veterinarian evaluated Running Bear by assessing his pulse, respiration, gut sounds and soundness. I breathed a sigh of relief when it was proclaimed that Running Bear passed the vet check. In the meantime, Russ did not wait for me but ran off ahead on the trail, and I recall that we never caught up to him again. This part of the race was easy; I simply rode my horse and felt relaxed. Well, let's say I was more relaxed than before. The last few miles of this race were a steep, twisty, rocky downhill trail, which slowed us down and made it impossible to catch my partner.

A super runner like Russ Kiernan can easily out-distance an equine on a downhill trail. I made sure to carefully take my horse slowly down this part of the route. When a trail is steep, rutted, and rocky it's easy for a horse to become lame, and I certainly didn't want to injure Running Bear. A horse is vulnerable to injury, especially tendons, on the downhills. Horses' front legs are long and spindly, making them injury-prone. Eventually, Running Bear and I safely arrived at the finish line where we found Russ waiting for us.

This race seemed pretty easy for me. I did some running and I didn't have to deal with big hills either going up or running down. It seemed that Running Bear and Russ did the hard work. As it turned out, we won the Pro-Am Division and came in seventh place overall! I was pleased with myself, and even more so with my horse.

I remembered sitting around after the race, talking to some of the other participants at the awards luncheon including Warren Hellman, Dan Barger, and Mark Rickman. As I got to know Dan and Mark, I found out they were world-class runners and Warren was one of the main sponsors of Ride & Tie. Russ Kiernan made this race easy for me and I was hooked but I didn't know it at that time. It had been a long time since I had so much fun, accompanied with the feeling of accomplishment.

My life changed dramatically after that day. I was separated from my wife, headed for divorce; I was vulnerable and definitely needed a change. I was competitive and I liked having fun. For me Ride & Tie was joyful, exciting and a new challenge.

In retrospect, I discovered that the competitors in Ride & Tie have aged through the years just like in other sports. The trend of the older athlete still in competition is very apparent, and I wanted to continue to become part of that phenomena.

Owning and taking care of a horse was therapeutic for me. I rode in the mornings before going into the office and riding became, thank goodness, an everyday occurrence. I worked long hours as a psycho-therapist and horseback riding, along with keeping a routine, helped me defend against work burn-out. It was important to my well-being, along with riding my Harley-Davidson motorcycle. I even joined the Fremont Hog Chapter and rode with the guys on the weekends.

Prior to this Ride & Tie life-changing event, my existence consisted of working and riding my horse and motorcycle for pleasure, not sport. I was looking for meaning in my life, only I didn't know it. I just knew something was missing. I was now able to set goals and again be com-petitive. My Ride & Tie experience added another significant dimen-sion to my being. I could focus, evaluate my running improvement, and create success and higher levels of aspiration. I was increasing my running distances, and conditioning myself and my horse. Little did I know at that time but I was about to find greater meaning in my life. Thank you, Russ Kiernan, for making that first Ride & Tie experience significant, exciting, meaningful and life-changing.

IV

Russ Kiernan: Dipsea Legend

Russ Kiernan is known as "Dipsea Legend." To the uninitiated it may seem like an odd title, but to the informed the title "Dipsea Legend" is spoken with reverence and admiration.

The Dipsea Race is the third oldest foot running race in the United States, and the oldest trail race in the U.S. It started in 1905 on a bet between members of the San Francisco Olympic Club, and the challenge was so exciting that they decided to make it a yearly affair. The year 2010 marked the 100th running of the event. Held every second Sunday in June, the Dipsea traverses 7.4 scenic, rugged miles from Mill Valley to Stinson Beach north of San Francisco, attracting thousands who vie for the maximum 1,500 entries.

Statistically speaking, Russ is around 6 feet tall, weighs about 145 pounds, and was born January 8, 1938. In addition to his Ride & Tie achievements, Russ has numerous awards and running-related accomplishments including the honor of being a three-time winner of the Dipsea (1998, 2002, 2005) and an 11-time winner of the Double Dipsea (a once-up and once-back race on the same trail as the Dipsea, doubling the mileage).

In 1946, Russ, his parents John and Gertrude, his two brothers Jack and Don, and sister Marie moved from Oakland, California, to a family member's house at 10th and Geary in San Francisco. About a year later, several of his cousins followed suit and joined the Kiernan family there. The entire clan lived in that house in the Richmond District of San Francisco until 1966 when the house burned to the ground. Adding to the tragedy, Russ also lost his father in the fire.

While growing up, Russ played basketball and baseball—typical team sports for boys of elementary and high school age. Illness forced him to miss part of high school, and as a result he didn't learn math very well. Actually, he didn't think that his schooling was all that terrific to begin with.

The one activity in which he excelled, however, was drinking at neighborhood bars, and as the years unfurled alcohol played a significant role in Russ's life. He started drinking as a freshman in high school, managed to get obnoxiously inebriated at his brother Jack's wedding, and was basically drunk more often than not. He believed that his father was an alcoholic and that heavy drinking was a commonplace pastime for certain family members and neighborhood locals.

After graduating from high school, Russ's life was unresolved and lacked direction. He literally didn't know what to do. One passing thought was to become a Merchant Marine. Thank goodness for his mother and brother Don's suggestion to Russ that he consider enrolling in a community college. Don had returned from military service and was attending a nearby community college, where he thought Russ could get some bearing and focus. Don told him what classes he should take, and the now guided Russ got in line and signed up for a full course load. After completing the requirements for an associate degree, Russ lent an ear as his brother proposed that he pursue a four-year degree, majoring in elementary education. Again, Russ listened intently and dutifully followed Don's advice. Don, who was four years older than Russ, was a good role model. Russ looked up to him and happily followed his guidance.

In the late 1950s Russ's brother Don became a cross-country running and swimming coach and a member of local running clubs. Accustomed to following in Don's footsteps, Russ started running with his mentor. It helped to have a partner who could assist with motivation, procuring the right equipment, and proper teaching techniques.

The Bay to Breakers Race in San Francisco is a running race, and the second oldest competition of its type in the U.S., surpassed in longevity only by the Boston Marathon. The Bay to Breakers Race is a 12k event, attended literally by tens of thousands of runners and supported by some 80,000 spectators, volunteers and staff on the day of the race. The route spans from the northeast end of town (the "bay" side) to the "breakers" of Ocean Beach, 7.46 miles away. Over the event's 100 years, it's estimated that 1.7 million participants have enjoyed this historic race, at whatever pace they chose. Competitors are an eclectic mixture of world-class determined runners and flamboyantly costumed participants out for an adventuresome stroll.

Russ ran 10 Bay to Breakers races from 1967 through 1987. He reflected, "I stopped doing them because it became a hassle with all the people who show up. Because of the enormous crowds, it becomes a nightmare at the start and as a result it's difficult to compete. And I like to compete."

As a young boy, Russ rode his bicycle along the Bay to Breakers course while attempting to keep up with competitor and five-time winner Kenny Moore. Russ quietly (and succinctly) reports, "He ran fast." That experience of peddling alongside a world-class runner thrilled Russ and resulted in a life-long impression.

Russ's first wife, Anita, died from hypertension in 1966 at the age of 25. As you recall, Russ also lost his father in 1966. It was in this significant year, at age 28, that Russ's illustrious running career started.

There is no doubt that there is a connection and a positive correlation between the loss of his father and wife, and the start of his running career. The direction of Russ's life took a huge turn. These major traumas resulted in Russ choosing a different and healthier path in life, as well as changes to his equilibrium and routine. There was now a shift in his habits and comfort level. Studies show that it is not uncommon for an individual to be in crisis, anxious, depressed, immersed in a troubled state, and then be able to pull together and turn the direction of their life around. Time and again individuals can and do just that, and refuse to surrender to the role of victim. For these individuals, the trauma of a negative valence changes into a positive life-fulfilling valence. The sport of running and the positive social interaction that accompanies it made the difference for Russ and he found a new, healthier family.

Then Russ met a teacher named Marilyn. They married in 1967 and moved to Mill Valley, north of San Francisco. He ran his first Dipsea in 1969 and has been running this race ever since. He missed the event in 1973 because he was in Europe, and again in 1976 and 1989 because of injuries.

In his endeavors to enter the world of competitive running, Russ remembers that he would venture to the local high school track to train, and watched as other runners around him worked out. He quickly discovered that these runners were fast, really fast. At first he would drive his car to the track, but after a while he would run from home to the track and then back, adding to his practice routine.

One day in 1971, long-distance runner Hans Roenau, who was born in Austria and grew up in Shanghai, invited Russ to run with the Saturday running group—the elite group. Russ made comments like, "I was in over my head," "these guys are fast," and "I'd better train." At that time, he was running on the track about four to five miles each session, maybe three miles in the hills, for a total of about fifteen to twenty miles a week. He's not exactly sure of those early distances, but he started running seriously in 1974 or 1975, racking up about thirty five to fifty miles per week. Russ confidently knew, "Now I can run with these guys." 'These guys' were all experienced Dipsea runners.

For Russ, training for the Dipsea begins the day after each yearly race. Barry Spitz, a Dipsea historian, predicted that Russ would win the 2009 Dipsea. Russ reflected about that particular race, "The week before the race I thought I had a chance to win. I felt okay, but I wasn't running as well as in the past." Earlier in the year Russ had a squamous cell skin cancer removed but developed an infection and was on medication. He finished the medication treatment a week before the race and realized that, "Running was more of a struggle. It was taking me longer to run the trails. I was slower and dragging." This assessment was a reflection of how Russ monitored himself, knew his body, employed both positive and negative reinforcement, and was extremely focused on his goal.

During the 2009 race, various thoughts ran through his head. "Can I do it?" "My times are slower," "It's tougher getting up these stairs," and "I should be able to hold them off." He had a nervous stomach and harbored considerable doubts. "I'm not going to be in the top ten. Maybe I can catch the runner ahead." He didn't, and wound up in 11th place.

As far as his nutritional program, Russ eats red meat, uses an Amway product called 'Neutral Light' and takes various nutrients such as a multivitamin, extra Vitamin C, calcium, magnesium, Vitamin B complex, rhodiola (an herb extract), and an energy drink with electrolytes.

For training purposes, Russ breaks the Dipsea Race into distance segments. He knows how much time each of these distances is supposed to take, and also factors in weather conditions. He'll take off from his training routine for three or four days before race day. Russ's typical training regimen consists of periodic limited speed work, and he consistently maintains positive thinking. He monitors how he feels in order to determine how far and how fast he runs that day, and eventually over the years, his goal has changed from finishing to winning.

Russ reports (with gratitude and admiration) that Jack Kirk, whom he met at the Dipsea, was his mentor and long-time friend. Jack, known as the "Dipsea Demon," was born in 1906 and died in 2007 at age 100. Jack was a colorful character and wonderfully eccentric; he ran all his races wearing rolled-down socks and a wool beanie. Russ remembers that Jack drove an old VW that served as his sleeping van as well as his office. After a race, Jack would hotwire his vehicle and unceremoniously drive away. He didn't have a key to his car, nor did he need one.

In 1930, at the age of 23, Jack ran his first Dipsea. He ran his last in 2003 at the age of 97. In 1997, he set the record for running in a single foot race for the most consecutive years when he surpassed Johnny Kelley's record of running the Boston Marathon. According to Russ, everybody who knew Jack had a distinct opinion of him. "You either liked him or disliked him. There was no neutral position."

Jack sent Russ letters which contained advice on how best to prepare for the Dipsea. He would say things like, "My philosophy of training is to not overly train. Save that super effort for the real race. When you are in good stairway shape, then without exercising too hard, try timing your stairway efforts and in case you don't know this, a downhill is just as important as an uphill. I inquired of the other runners as to what was the most difficult section of the course. The consensus was the stairs. Do not be afraid to win again." In the Dipsea, there are 671 stairs to navigate. In his later years, Jack wisely told Russ, "You don't die; you go to the 672nd stair."

At Jack's funeral, his friend Ron Goode presented the eulogy. He shared that Jack claimed he first started building those strong legs when he lived in Martinez, California, in 1925. "Jack lived down the street from the DiMaggio's. He and his brothers would throw rocks at the DiMaggio house and wait for them to respond." They would run as fast as they could to escape the retaliating rocks thrown back at them. One might say that the Kirk brothers helped develop the strong arms of the famous baseball-playing DiMaggio brothers. Ron also said that later in life Jack boasted that he was the only Mariposa, California, resident to serve time in three jails. In actuality, Jack would simply (but emphatically) state, "I want my day in court."

At one point in time, Ron had asked Jack which was the hardest run he ever tackled. Without blinking or pausing, Jack replied, "The Double Diablo!" When asked about the Bay to Breakers, Jack commented, "There were thousands of runners, and they put me up front with the fastest runners. I would run like I never ran before straight to the first doorway, grab the doorframe and wait for an hour. Then I rocked with the rest of the group."

As the years unfolded in Jack's fascinating life, he was asked about the secret of his longevity. Without missing a beat, he responded with a twinkle in his eye, "Keep breathing."

In 1989 Russ ran the Dipsea course with Jack Kirk and Charlie Richeisen, a former Dipsea winner who had recorded Jack's tales about his many Dipsea races. As Russ accompanied Charlie and Jack during one of the interview sessions, "Jack showed us all the old shortcuts on the trail," remembers Russ, "all the while identifying wildflowers and other plants along the route. He was a wealth of information and advice. We got back to his old Volkswagen bug, which he had slept in the night before. He refused to come in for even a drink of water. He hotwired his car and left for his home in Mariposa. Jack was 82 at the time. He continued to send me letters of advice and encouragement on winning the Dipsea."

Russ Kiernan reported that he successfully incorporated Jack's training techniques. Russ had turned running the Dipsea into a science and had broken down the race into nine categories ranging from the first step, to the finish. He'd created a spreadsheet of columns starting with his 1975 run based on a 60-minute pace, to the year 2000 with a 70-minute pace. In this chart, Russ configured the running times for each segment of the trail, with his timed pace at different ages. This training technique kept track of his times at specific points of the trail and helped him predict his time at the finish. Not surprisingly, Russ was happy to share his training technique with others.

Russ's role models included Jack Kirk, the "Dipsea Demon," and his wife Marilyn, who supports him in all his running events. His goals, as he stated in 2009, include, "Continuing to run a time equal to my age in the Dipsea and to win the race again within the next three years." He keeps a log of his best recent performances, personal records and other running-related accomplishments.

Russ has also competed in Ride & Tie events, with 28 completions in the World Ride & Tie Championships, complemented by many Top Ten finishes. The 2009 World Ride & Tie Championship was held at Cuneo Creek in Northern California; a competition described by Russ Kiernan as, "The ride from hell!" When he arrived at Cuneo Creek, Russ didn't have a partner or a horse for the event, and most teams were already formed. Luckily Don Betts told Russ he knew of a horse with a partner—Rachel Toor and steed "Pip." Russ's wife Marilyn asked Don about the horse; his reply was, "He's crazy." On race day, Russ was mounted on Pip and just before the start he realized that the horse was 'full of it.' Regardless of what he did, the horse would not settle down. Russ was a terrific runner, and typically his first position at Ride & Tie races was to start out on foot. This time was different and he knew he was in for the ride of his life when the horse blasted out at the start of the race. The race started fine since they were going uphill in the beginning. The plan was for him to ride about a mile and then get off the horse and pass the tie rope to an individual on the ground for a "hand tie." He thought he was still okay, because he was then on the ground and running. Rachel and Pip caught up to him in about 10 minutes, and they switched positions. Again he mounted Pip and rode for another four to five minutes, dismounted and tied the horse to a tree limb. He continued running and made more horse exchanges with Rachel. Now he was racing the downhill section of the race, and he quickly realized that Pip was indeed more than he could handle. His desperate thought was, "This was going to be the last day of my life."

Russ remarked, "This crazy beast ran away with me three times before I flew off of him on a sharp downhill turn." The horse continued to run downhill full-bore. Thank goodness Russ was wearing a helmet. Hurting, he began hobbling down the trail. A few miles later, he crossed paths with a hiker who told him that his horse was tied to a tree ahead. When he reached up to untie the horse, he asked himself, "Am I nuts?" Regardless of how honest his answer was, he got on anyway. Both of them made it down the rest of the hill and eventually arrived at the veterinary checkpoint. His partner Rachel was waiting there. They had just finished seventeen miles, so he ate and drank and headed out on foot for Loop 2. Rachel was in front on Pip. This was a 12-mile loop—about five miles uphill and about five miles downhill. At each end of the loop, for about a mile, the trail was relatively flat. The horse was more controllable, but "I felt like a rag doll," said Russ.

Rachel and the horse made a wrong turn on Loop 2, so when Russ arrived at the next vet check, there was no horse or partner. A mandatory rule in Ride & Tie competitions is that the partners—the human ones—must make a rider exchange at each vet check. So Russ could not continue; he had to be in the saddle for the next stretch. About 30 minutes later, the rest of his team arrived. Rachel started running on Loop 3 while Russ took the horse through the mandatory veterinary check and then mounted up. Loop 3 had a long uphill, and then a downhill with switchbacks. They had to cross a creek before reaching the flat trail. Although extremely tired, Russ thought this section went well even though he had never ridden this far on any other Ride & Tie. And then, he went off Pip again, hitting the dirt hard. In a repeat performance, Pip took off trotting down the trail, sans human. Luckily there was a competitor ahead of Pip who grabbed the reins and held this wild beast. Eventually, Russ got back on the horse and made it to the finish line. He said, "After more than six hours of hell, I was never so happy to see a finish line!"

It's clear that Russ is extremely focused. He is persistent, and takes an intelligent approach to any activity that provides him with both personal satisfaction and meaning to his life. He is competitive, a high achiever, employs self-reinforcement, and keeps within his ability to know himself. He is a successful, important part of the running community. He looks to the future, continues to set realistic goals, and loves playing like a young person. For these reasons my first Ride & Tie, with Russ as my competent partner, was relatively easy.

The Dipsea cross-country trail-running event begins in downtown Mill Valley. Runners traverse 671 stairs leading up to the side of Mt. Tamalpais, then pass through Muir Woods National Monument in Mount Tamalpais State Park, wind through the Golden Gate National Recreation Area and finally end at the quaint village of Stinson Beach. Among the many challenges facing the participants is the uneven footing of the trail on this single-track foot path, and the steep terrain that features about 2200 feet of elevation gain and loss over the course.

This race has a handicap system that often produces younger or older winners. Most participants, with the exception of the "scratch" runners, are given a head start based on their age and gender. The oldest and youngest runners are given up to a 25-minute advantage over the fastest competitors, making it virtually possible for any age group to produce a race winner. It's a popular race; as many as 3,000 people apply for entry each year. But the field of competitors is limited to 1,500 due to safety and environmental considerations. This makes it difficult for many people to get accepted into the race. There was no official race in 1932 and 1933 due to economic conditions, nor were there races from 1942 through 1945 because of World War II.

Being a three-time winner of the Dipsea (1998, 2002, and 2005); 11-time winner of the Double Dipsea; 26 top-10 Dipsea finishes; and 29 Black Shirts for finishing in the top 35 certainly puts Russ in the Dipsea Hall of Fame. But Russ also gives back to his community. He continues to be the coach for the Tamalpais summer youth program, and is assistant coach at the Mill Valley Middle School. I don't know anyone more committed to pursuing excellence than Russ.

V

My Second Ride & Tie: The World Championship

My second Ride & Tie event, the world championship in 1997, was in beautiful Fort Bragg along the coast in Northern California. My partner was Paul Robinson, who was recommended by Robert Eichstaedt. The four of us; Robert, Paul, my horse Running Bear, and I met before the big event in Marin County for a practice Ride & Tie near Mount Tamalpais. The trail was literally in Russ Kiernan's backyard.

I remember very clearly Paul saying that I was not going to get off as easy as I did at the Quicksilver Ride & Tie with Russ as my partner. In this championship race with Paul as my partner, I was going to have to pull my load, which translated to a lot of running. The course at Fort Bragg was 35 tough miles. Robert told me that one way to train for the championship was to run twice a day. Oh great, just what I wanted to hear. Well, I didn't run twice a day and I paid for it dearly during and after the race.

During those early days, my Ride & Tie outfit consisted of a cotton T-shirt, Levi cutoffs, baseball cap, and running shoes. I quickly learned the problem with wearing Levi cutoffs: chaffed legs, resulting from friction with the saddle stirrup leathers (the looped leather strips that attach the stirrups to the actual saddle). You can't even imagine how much pain those chaffed areas caused with every stride of the horse!

Always on a quest to better my comfort and performance, I experimented with various options like high-rise soccer socks, but I didn't like them because they didn't stay up. I even thought of wearing pantyhose (gasp!) to protect my legs. The chaffing problem eventually was solved by wearing synthetic running tights (the material doesn't shift, fold or rub) and placing a comfy sheepskin over the saddle. I also learned why wearing cotton clothing is not the best choice, based on what happens with sweat, evaporation, wicking and wrinkles. A synthetic-blend running shirt, tights, and running shoes designed specifically for trails worked so much better, which kept me so much happier! I also learned what to drink and eat during these events, which can make the difference between finishing with a smile and finishing with a grimace. Products like Gatorade, GU Electrolyte Brew, Cytomax, GU, and Power Bars worked well. Paying attention to electrolytes and what food is readily and easily digestible is an important part of a running strategy. And I found that experienced Ride & Tie participants were extremely helpful and willing to share their tips for success, and I was grateful to learn from them.

At the Fort Bragg Ride & Tie, I started to park my truck and horse trailer when I saw Steve Shaw waving at me so he could tell me where to park. It was an interesting crossroad when I first met Steve. Years before, my wife at the time, and some other friends and I went on a motorcycle excursion up the northern coast of California to Fort Bragg. The woman who agreed to look after our dogs, cats, and horses while we were gone asked a friend to join her as she cared for our animals and property. Her friend was Eileen, Steve Shaw's wife. Eileen was killed in an automobile accident shortly afterwards. I did not know Eileen or Steve at that time, but it seemed rather Kismet-like to see Steve at Fort Bragg. Years later, I talked with Steve about that coincidence. It's amazing how the groups of people in these sports all intertwine, and seemingly everything comes full circle. It's that 'tribe' feeling that is such a significant part of what attracts me to these sports and these folks. I think, as a culture, we have lost that feeling of community, and finding it here filled a hole in my life.

The temperature was creeping up to triple digits, and I did some walking during the race, a lot of walking. Eventually, Paul, Running Bear and I completed the event. We did not win any awards nor did we finish in the top ten, but we were pleased about finally seeing the finish line on the horizon, and having bragging rights about completing this tough race. I don't know how long the event took us, but I remember that I was out on the trail running (okay, walking), for a long, long time.

Here's an honest admission: One thing that stands out in my mind about this competition is the difficulty I had getting out of bed the next morning. My lower back was sore overall, peppered with occasional acute shooting pains somewhat akin to what I imagine it's like to be shot with an arrow. My entire body seemed beat up. I was so relieved to be able to drive home without incident, fearing that my pain would overtake my driving skills! That was a huge check-in with reality, an in-your-face experience of Ride & Tie. Bottom line: it's damned hard. It became painfully (literally and figuratively) clear that I had a lot of work ahead to get Running Bear and me in better trail shape.

I began to run more seriously after that Ride & Tie Championship. My horse seemed to be in better condition than me, and was able to comfortably handle the endurance and distance for Ride & Tie competitions. Now all I had to do was to improve my stamina.

My second world championship Ride & Tie was in 1998 and held at Donner Summit in Northern California. The Sunday prior to this big race was when I hurt my back while getting my truck and camper ready. I was hooking up my horse trailer to my rig. I backed up my 1-ton Ford truck and was almost perfectly aligned with the tongue and receiver of the horse trailer. Notice, I said 'almost perfectly aligned.' So, looking at my situation I could do one of two things. I could pull the truck forward and then back to better the alignment or I could attempt to manually move the tongue of the horse trailer. Unfortunately, I chose the latter. In doing so, I hurt my lower back. So that night I made two more huge mistakes. First, I did some sit-ups on the hardwood floor. Don't ask me why I did sit-ups. Second, I applied heat to my lower back. At the time, I knew very little about dealing with injuries.

As I couldn't walk, I literally crawled up the steps to my second-floor bedroom and I couldn't get out of bed the next morning. I called my son Geoffrey and asked him to come over. And then I called my friend Gary Lindahl, a physical therapist, whose office was across the street from mine. Luckily, he was there, answered the phone, and instructed me on the technique of sitting up on the edge of the bed and then getting to my feet. He told me to come to his office prior to my appointments and he would help me get through the day. I found that when I was on my feet I felt better. Walking seemed to be the best therapy. I did not want to go into back spasms again. Later that morning I managed to drive to Gary's office.

Gary treated me and I felt better. He instructed me in taking Advil, icing, getting a proper back support, and walking before the next day's treatment. I then proceeded to my office for a day and evening of psychotherapy. I remember that I stood up while my clients sat during our sessions. It was easier to stand than to sit. The rest of the week was pretty much the same. I would go on long walks, then see Gary for treatment, and then stand during the psychotherapy sessions. I called my Ride & Tie partner Steve Anderson and told him what I was going through. I suggested that he come over Friday and we would drive to Donner and hope that I would be able to ride on Saturday. I mentioned that he would do the driving, and we would stop about every hour so I could get out and stretch my back. We finally arrived at our destination and Steve did all the work in getting ready for Saturday's big event. I still didn't know whether I could get on Running Bear's back. I felt miserable but I wanted to compete.

Saturday morning came. I asked Steve to saddle up my horse for me and then I was actually able to get on Running Bear's back. I told Steve that I would do my best in running and riding but I didn't know what to expect. I had visions of myself lying on the trail with my back in spasms. I could be called by some a 'nutcase;' maybe I needed psychotherapy.

At the start, all the horses and riders were in a large open space. It became clear that all these horses would have to converge quickly on a very narrow trail. I was lucky that I was not thrown from my horse and trampled by fast charging horses. I hung on, and what a rush! My heart was pounding, blood flowing; what a thrill. Ride & Tie was a fun sport.

I quickly found out that after getting off my horse I felt better while running. I didn't fall to the ground and my back didn't go into spasms.

Trail running seemed to be the right therapy for me. I was pleased that I was able to complete this race and that my physical condition did not get worse.

Then the awards ceremony followed. That was awful because I was sitting in the chair for much of the time, and I was still hurting when I wasn't running. We left for home shortly thereafter, and the rest of the day was a blur.

The 1999 world championship Ride & Tie was held in Klamath Falls, Oregon. I was fine physically and teamed up with Steve Anderson again, and with a horse that I borrowed from Peter Rich. I was looking for another horse to purchase and remembered my friend who had a ranch adjacent to Tilden Park in the Berkeley hills. I spent some time there riding and evaluating horses to purchase. I was fortunate in that I was permitted to take this horse for the Ride & Tie championship in Oregon. The ride went well, but due to some advice my equestrian friends gave, I chose not to purchase the horse I rode.

To help reach my goals, I ran a trail half-marathon with Steve Anderson, my Ride & Tie partner at the tough Lake Chabot competition. That half-marathon went fairly well. Then I started running longer distances on a bike and horse path adjacent to the horse stable where my horse died. This flat trail had human drinking water along the way and was about 20 miles in distance. I was approaching marathon-length distance, and was actually running the hills now. I was definitely improving!

Between 1997 and 1999, I participated in a number of Ride & Tie events. I ran my first ultra run, a 50K at Lake Chabot. I remember asking other runners about the cut-off time; their consistent response was, "You're doing fine—don't worry about it." In addition to worrying, I wound up with horrible blisters on both feet. I felt exhausted for at least a couple of weeks, but I was still alive!

During this time I met a man who was at least 10 years older than me; Bob Edwards. He was a real character, a good runner, good horseman, and a breeder of Arabian horses. He had an incredible spirit of determination, framed by a wonderfully ruddy face that looked as though it was a road map of adventures he had joyfully conquered. He really knew the Ride & Tie community, and through him I got to know a lot of people in this sport. Mind you, my initial impression of Ride & Tie people was that they are not very friendly and there seemed to be a lot of cliques. But after a while, and especially because of Bob, I began to fit in much better.

Bob and I did many events together, including a Ride & Tie called the Bloomfield Boogie located at the Skillman campground near Nevada City, in California's Gold Rush country. Bob drove in from Arroyo Grande where he lived, and we both arrived on Friday in time for tale-swapping and a good dinner. We unfolded our camp chairs, sat down, and planned for Saturday's race. He brought his mare, Fancy Belle, for the event and I got on her that evening to get some sense of her personality and what she was like. I don't remember how we finished in the event, but the important thing is, it was the start of a long-term friendship.

An extraordinary raconteur, Bob would regale those gathered about him with stories about horses, running, Ride & Tie, and growing up as a kid in Utah. Bob had entered the Tevis that year, and I helped crew for him and his horse. Neighbor Sandy, and Bob's roommate Diane, were also entered. I drove to Auburn, which is the ending point for the ride, and met Dennis Burkett there, who was a good friend of Bob's. We stayed at Dennis's home, and then on Saturday morning, Dennis and I drove to Robinson Flat (36 miles into the 100-mile event and the first one-hour veterinary checkpoint on the trail) to crew for the three riders.

Let me give you a brief overview of what Robinson Flat is like. Robinson Flat is in the U.S. Forest Service domain, a small meadow area surrounded by logging roads and places where loggers 'skid' their loads for pickup. It's an amazingly beautiful, quiet site, far away from civilization and at an altitude of 6730 feet. For 363 days out of the year, it's a peaceful and serene spot in the wilderness. During Tevis, however, it's teeming with life, action and drama. The horses and riders have come 36 miles from the start, up Squaw Peak and over the original Emigrant Trail, past Watson's Monument, through bogs, over slick granite, and along the rocky crest of the Sierra Nevada Mountains. Most riders have two or three people crewing for them at Robinson, plus a myriad of veterinarians, pulse and respiration personnel (who check the horses), photographers, dogs, WSTF officials and the WSTF Cup Committee, journalists, horseshoers, Forest Service officials, water trucks, hay stations, timers, horse trailer transport—it's as though the forest at Robinson Flat has literally exploded with people and supplies. A conservative estimate would be that some 1,000 people arrive to serve the needs of 250 riders and horses. The excitement builds as people line the trail, craning their necks to see if they can see their rider coming in. The rider dismounts, the saddle is pulled, dust is wiped from the rider's eyes, timer cards are swooped up, and then it's a calculated process of presenting the horse to the veterinary staff who then evaluate the ability of the horse to progress down the trail. The ensuing mandatory hour hold is filled with hydrating rider and steed, filling guts with hay, grain, bran mash, electrolytes and supplements for the horses, and sandwiches, cookies, fruit, electrolytes and whatever fits the fancy of the rider. Hands appear to massage the horse and the rider, keeping muscles supple and warm. A swift 60 minutes pass, and saddle and bridle are reattached to the horse. The rider now has clean socks on, and it's down the trail for those lucky enough to have passed veterinary criteria.

From there, we drove to Michigan Bluff (62.5 miles from the start of the competition) to crew and meet the riders. Michigan Bluff is typically a sleepy little burg of about 40 people (except on Tevis and Western States), perched high above the North Fork of the American River. It was a booming place for gold miners in the late 1840s through the 1850s, replete with brothel, hotel, and a merchandise store owned by Leland Stanford of Stanford University fame. The town continues to be charming, bolstered by dedicated souls determined to live an unconventional life, and by a working gold mine called the Big Gun Mine.

Upon arriving in Michigan Bluff, the horses and riders had pulled up out of El Dorado Canyon where temperatures can reach 120 degrees, a tough haul for even the fittest competitors.

After Michigan Bluff, we drove to Foresthill (68 miles into the ride and the second one-hour veterinary checkpoint) to help the horses and riders. Foresthill is also a remnant of the Gold Rush Days, and has its own charm and character. At 3225 feet, the vet check was at an old milling site, flat and spacious. The local school had a booth selling ice cream, and you could buy a pretty darned good hamburger right at the vet check. Most riders arrived as the sun was setting, making the temperature much more bearable, with many horses getting their 'second wind' after some rest and recuperation. At Foresthill, both Bob and Diane were pulled out of the competition—their horses did not meet the strict veterinary requirements. Now only Sandy remained in the competition. Dennis, Bob, and Diane went to the Gold Country Fairgrounds in Auburn to wait for Sandy at the finish line.

I went back to Dennis's house because I had planned to drive to Redding in Northern California on Sunday to look at a horse to buy. As it turned out, Sandy got pulled and I didn't go to Redding. This Tevis experience gave me a great overview of the race and the complexity of the logistics necessary to compete. This particular ride is a real hassle for crews because of the great driving distance from the start point of Robie Park, where everyone camps the day before the ride, to the first crewing point at Robinson Flat. After the horses and riders leave the start at Robie Park (at 5:00 a.m.), crews have one heck of a drive to meet the riders at Robinson Flat. The horses and riders traverse 36 miles to Robinson, but the crews have to drive 115 miles to the same point and it takes a solid three hours or more to drive there. Obviously one has to plan and organize for these extraordinary logistics. Seeing the Tevis first-hand as part of a crew motivated me to begin thinking about riding this event.

Bob Edwards was an excellent runner. He ran ultras and planned to run the Western States 100. He committed to participating in a three-day Western States training event, held every Memorial Day weekend. Participants run about 75 miles over the three days, going from Robinson Flat to Auburn along the Run trail, which is almost identical to the Tevis Trail. Training event participants can't start at Squaw Valley where the Run officially starts, however, because it's too early in the year and there's too much snow on the trail.

I told Bob I would meet him at the Foresthill campsite and run the second day with him from Foresthill to White Oak Flat. At approximately 16 miles into the run, I was in front of Bob and his friend at an aid station, eating and drinking, and feeling pretty good about what I'd accomplished. Remember, Bob ran about 32 miles the previous day. Then, I looked over to the trail and saw Bob running by with a shit-eating grin on his face, laughing the whole time. I had to get moving!

The next three-mile section of the trail was all uphill and I made sure I got in front of Bob. Now I had a good overview of the Western States Trail, with a vantage point for both human and equestrian.

These two events are monumental and prestigious in the endurance and ultra running worlds; the granddaddies of them all. They are considered to be the ultimate competitions, and I now had them firmly planted in my subconscious, just waiting to come to the surface.

VI

History of the Tevis

The year 2000 was momentous in my life. My new girlfriend Judy and I were living in Cool, California, in the Sierra foothills between Sacramento and Lake Tahoe; just a few miles from Coloma where gold was initially discovered in 1848, prompting the historic Gold Rush. Tom and Laura Christofk and Jerome Beauchamp, Ride & Tie competitors, lived in this Gold Country area and were an influence to us moving to Cool.

After our move I found out the third annual Maui Marathon was being held on the 19th of March. Why not participate in that marathon as part of a vacation? I had not run a marathon to this point, but I had one 50K run under my belt. I certainly remembered that one, complete with miserable blisters. I painfully remembered how sore and awful I hurt afterwards. One concern that I had was the humid weather in Hawaii that time of year. My training in Northern California consisted of running in cold, wet weather, on muddy single track trails. How could I prepare for heat and humidity while training in a Northern California winter? I remember Tom telling me, "Don't worry about it, you will do just fine." Maybe Tom knew something I didn't.

The event started near the airport and it seemed like there were thousands of runners; I was amazed. I looked up and saw signs with numbers posted. One sign said something like 3 to 3-1/2 hours, and I don't remember which group I got into, but I wasn't in front. I entered the grouping that I thought was appropriate, but I wasn't sure.

It was an early morning start, which I liked because the weather was rather cool at that hour. The race began and it seemed like thousands of runners were ahead of me. I wasn't thrilled with my position, but after a short while I got to the main road that paralleled the ocean. This road led the runners to the finish line at the Kaanapali district, with aid stations at every mile point. Automobiles and trucks full of people screaming in enthusiastic support traversed the marathon route. This event was an annual fundraiser, so it was a big deal on the island.

The temperature was warm, but the humidity was not stifling. I was tired when I got to Lahaina and was glad it was near the end of the race. I found that I had enough reserve to get to the finish at Kaanapali. I crossed the finishing line feeling great. My four-hour-45-minute time was not spectacular, but it was okay.

With this marathon out of the way, I could now put my energy and focus on the Tevis, which was my primary goal. By completing a marathon and the 50K, I had accomplished two of my running goals, which fit in nicely with my desire to do well in Ride & Tie. I felt better about my running ability because I could now see that I was improving. I wanted to be able to run the mileage of an entire Ride & Tie event (only if necessary, of course!). My thinking was that I wanted to be able to do what my horse did on foot, only no one would be on my back.

Let's return to the fall of 1999, before moving to Cool. I purchased a new horse in August, a half-Arabian, half-Quarter Horse. He was a roan gelding who I quickly named 'Red Raider' after the Oakland Raiders. I completed one endurance ride in the fall of 1999, the Lake Sonoma 50, and I'm glad that Raider and I did fine. That was my first 50-mile endurance ride and I was very pleased. I talked with Tom Christofk about my Tevis goal for the year 2000. To prepare for the Tevis, Tom suggested that I ride the Derby Ditch 50 in Nevada, the 50-mile ride at Whiskey Town in California, and the NASTR 75-mile ride in Nevada.

Tom, Tony Brickel and I charged along on training rides on the Tevis trail, riding at a fast clip from Foresthill to Poverty Bar and back, approximately 40 miles of single track trail with plenty of elevation change. Our second training ride, more difficult because of steep canyons, went from Foresthill to the swinging bridge (at the bottom of the canyon where the North Fork of the Middle Fork of the American River flows) and then back. We rode hard and fast. On that ride, I remember a runner by the name of Ann Trason running toward us in her own training run. Ann is a world-class runner and was the first woman finisher in the last 13 Western States 100 runs. No woman can beat her, and only a few men. She is awesome, and there is no one like her. Tom apparently knew her and struck up a conversation. Just behind her was runner Emma Davies from the San Francisco Bay Area. I met Emma while running and conditioning my horse at an East Bay Regional Park called Sunol. She recognized me and we had a brief conversation. Little did I know she would finish second to Ann two years later in the 2002 Western States Run.

The Western States Endurance Run begins at Squaw Valley (site of the 1960 Olympics) at the entrance to the ski slope and continues to the finish line at Placer High School in Auburn. This race is a one-day, 100-mile endurance run. Incidentally, Ann's finishing time in the 2002 race was 18 hours 16 minutes and 26 seconds, while Emma Davies finished in 18 hours 32 minutes and 17 seconds. These running times are incredible! I was not consciously thinking about running Western States at that point.

The Tevis is a 100-mile one-day endurance ride that begins at Robie Park near Truckee (north of Lake Tahoe) and ends at the fairgrounds in Auburn. The Tevis is rich in history and characters, and I'd like to share a bit of history about the ride and the man who started it. The following information is found in Bill G. Wilson's book, "Challenging the Mountains: The Life and Times of Wendell T. Robie."

In 1955, the Reno Gazette Journal had an article describing, "Some gentlemen from Auburn are attempting a one-day 100-mile ride out of Tahoe City." Five riders; Nick Mansfield, William Patrick, Pat Sewell, Richard Highfield, and Wendell Robie said they could ride over 9000 feet of summit, go through deep canyons, and follow a trail that no other horsemen had traveled on such a ride. This ride had a lot of unknowns. One major question was, could a horseback rider travel and cover 100 miles in a day?

Robie claimed that organizing the event would bring new home and property owners to Auburn and give valuable publicity to the town

(Robie was a businessman in Auburn—he was into lumber, real estate, and later started a bank). He quoted the Vermont organizers of a 100-mile Green Mountain trail ride, who claimed that people keep fit by riding horseback. He also quoted Winston Churchill's famous phrase, "The outside of a horse is good for the inside of a man."

Robie was influenced by pioneer Bob Watson, who was the last constable of Tahoe City. One of Watson's missions in life was to re-establish the original Emigrant Trail over the Sierra crest. Long lost to overgrowth and lack of use, the trail was used by Native Americans as part of their seasonal migratory route, as well as gold miners in the late 1840s and early 1850s that traversed this rugged trail in their search for instant riches. Later on in the 1850s, the trail was also used by those leaving California in search for silver in the Comstock Lode in Nevada. Watson's quest to redefine the trail was a proud endeavor, and he en-listed like-spirits in finding the trail, including Wendell Robie and a group of Auburn men who belonged to the Native Sons of the Golden West. In one of their trail-marking journeys in 1935, they took along a movie camera and captured the adventures of their ride, including pack horses breaking loose and scattering their goods over mountain ridges. In addition to finding and marking the entire trail, when he was in his 70s Bob Watson erected a shrine dedicated to all the pioneers who had traveled this trail. The edifice was later named Watson's Monument; located at the top of Emigrant Pass, and topped with an American flag that all the runners and riders pass by during their events.

In conjunction with the first 100-mile ride in 1955, Robie encour-aged men and women to make the same ride over the course of three days. The participants would cover 35 miles the first day, 38 miles a second day and 27 miles the final day. Ever the quintessential busi-nessman, Robie created the Western States Trail Foundation to oversee all these new ideas and events. He organized the three-day event as a "holiday on horseback", supported by printed brochures, maps, secre-taries, caterers, etc.

Robie's ride, officially called the Western States 100-Mile One-Day Ride, began at four o'clock in the morning. To protect the horses during the ride, they would all be examined at mandatory veterinary checkpoints. The veterinarians were from the school of veterinary medicine at the University of California, Davis. The first (and only) horse to be pulled by the vets on that historic day was Dick Highfield's horse. He was pulled at Robinson Flat, because he was lame, according to the vet. Rider Nick Mansfield was carrying an extra 60 pounds of food and horseshoes in his saddlebags. That poor horse had to haul all that extra weight. The vets, thank goodness, took his pack at Red Star Ridge, located before Robinson Flat. Mansfield, who went on to finish this 100-mile ride an admirable 16 times, actually rode from Reno to the start of the first 100-mile ride in 1955, adding another 40 miles to his 100-mile ride on Buffalo Bill. This horse finished the ride 11 times in his career; one of only five horses from 1955 to 2010 to finish the ride 10 times or more.

Even though Sewell and Patrick were much younger, they and their horses were exhausted during the ride. After leaving Foresthill, about 60 or so miles into the event, a young man named Harold Jay greeted them with, "Follow me and I'll guide you the rest of the way." The riders arrived at the Gold Country Fairgrounds in Auburn around 4:05 a.m. Sunday morning, after 22 hours and 45 minutes of riding. Unfortunately, these four riders did not get official riding time statistics. Remember how fast the two women covered 100 miles? The last 40 miles on the trail covered by the four men was in complete darkness. Darkness is not an issue for the horse since they have fairly good night vision. Otherwise, the ride would be impossible because of the dangerous trail and the fact that if the horse fell, there's a chance that both horse and rider could die. This is a single-track trail, not straight, with many hazardous spots and the American River far below the trail's edge.

Robie realized that he started an event that would likely continue as long as men bonded with their horses. He believed that this event was too much of a real challenge for super horsemen not to participate. This was the ride of a lifetime, following the historic Western States Trail over the Sierra. This trail varied in elevation from 8774 feet at Emigrant Pass to 12,000 feet at the finish line in Auburn.

Robie wrote letters to newspapers, magazines, and congressmen, and gave public talks everywhere. He made arrangements with the school of veterinary medicine at UC Davis and had veterinarians at the ride to protect the horses. To combat criticism from many riding groups and the humane society, he had his head veterinarian, Dr. Richard Barsaleau, counter their arguments.

The ride, even though its official name is Western States 100-Day 100-Mile Ride, is commonly known as The Tevis, and the award for the first place winner is the Tevis Cup which was first awarded in 1959 (the first ride was in 1955). The cup was named in honor of Lloyd Tevis, an adventuresome pioneer who came to California in a covered wagon in 1849 in search of gold. In true entrepreneurial spirit, Lloyd became the president of Wells Fargo & Co. from 1872 to 1892. The Tevis Cup was established as a perpetual trophy by his grandsons Will, Gordon, and Lloyd Tevis.

In 1964, Richard Barsaleau, DVM, was the key person in establishing an award for the horse to cross the finish line in the most superior physical condition. Even though Dr. Barsaleau wanted only the first five horses to be considered for this award, it was decided that the field should consist of the first 10 horses judged by a veterinary examining committee.

Louis Haggin of Versailles, Kentucky, donated the Haggin Cup to be awarded to that one special horse in superior physical condition. Louis's grandfather, James Ben Ali Haggin, had been Lloyd Tevis's business partner both in a San Francisco law practice (1853) and with Wells Fargo & Co. (Haggin was vice-president). The two pioneers had met in the gold fields in their quest for the "big strike." After being contacted by Lloyd Tevis (grandson of cup honoree), Louis Haggin agreed to donate the James Ben Ali Haggin Cup in honor of his grandfather, who was also a breeder of fine Thoroughbred horses. In fact, one of Haggin's horses, Ben Ali, won the Kentucky Derby in 1886.

The first Haggin Cup went to Paige Harper's horse, Keno, in 1964. Robie had the Haggin Cup inscribed with: "Kindness to animals despite adverse pressure is the mark of a man." The Haggin Cup is very coveted, and it's believed that when Robie won this award in 1965 on his stallion Siri, he was more proud of that honor than in coming in first overall (he won the ride in 1955, 1956, 1957, 1958). Robie, a stalwart soul, had a sign in his office that read, "Life is a mystery to be lived, not a problem to be solved."

Biologist Fred Jones was a personal friend of Robie's, and during the time of their friendship was appointed Director of the California Department of Parks and Recreation in March 1965 by Gov. Pat Brown. Fred inherited numerous boards and commissions, one of which was the Riding and Hiking Trails Advisory Committee. Wendell Robie was very active on this board and as a result Fred became acquainted with him.

Fred spent many summers in the early 1950s riding pack stock in the Sierra Nevada Mountains out of Owens Valley to conduct deer studies in three areas, so he was familiar with long rides. He heard of the Tevis Cup, and it caught his interest. He was even more curious because one of his friends at UC Berkeley was none other than Lloyd Tevis (grandson of Lloyd of Wells Fargo fame), who is a black sheep in the family because he became a biologist instead of following his family's banking business. Fred was game to try the 100-mile ride, and his only problem was that he needed to borrow a strong horse.

One of the riders in Wendell's group was a man who Fred knew from the California state government. What Fred didn't know was that Wendell assigned this man to recruit Fred as a ride contestant. One day Fred and this man sat next to each other on a plane to Los Angeles, and Fred decided to hit him up for the loan of a horse. Each of them worked the other to their mutual benefit.

About three weeks before the hundred mile ride, Fred got a Quarter Horse named Buck that had been out to pasture for a couple of years. Buck was turned out with a couple hundred other horses because he had hurt a rider in a rodeo. Paige Harper, another of Wendell's friends who Fred knew as a result of being on the advisory committee, met Fred at Folsom Lake one evening for an introduction to Buck and an initial training ride to Auburn. Since Buck hadn't been in the trailer before, Paige unloaded him with a bit of clatter. Paige saddled Buck and told Fred to mount up and trot the horse around the asphalt parking lot until he got his horse ready to ride. Buck did his thing—he got his head down and started bucking. Fred decided to step off at the low point, but got tossed backwards, landed on his butt with both hands splat on the asphalt. Buck pranced around until Paige got him under control. Paige told Fred to get back on, pull the reins tight so the horse's nose was against his neck, then pull hard to the left, kick him in the ribs and let him run around the parking lot. Paige then headed through the gate and up the hill with Fred and Buck following at a trot all the way until they reached Auburn some 25 to 30 miles up the trail.

The next morning Fred's back was so stiff he had a hard time getting up. He bought a Velcro corset and strapped it on. Fred then arranged for a trainer to ride Buck every day at a place in Newcastle where Dru Barner kept her horse Chagitai. Dru was Wendell's assistant at his bank, Heart Federal Savings and Loan, in Auburn and a very competent rider. In fact, she was the first woman to ever win the Tevis, which she did in 1961 on Chagitai in a riding time of 13:02.

Fred rode Buck every weekend on one of Wendell's long training rides. On one 50-mile run, a group mounted up at Squaw Valley and rode about 25 miles to the turnaround point. Wendell's modus operandi was to not stop at all. Fred planned on a bit of lunch and some rest, but it was not to be. So Fred munched on his sandwich and guzzled some water as they trotted along. Buck and Fred fell behind the group, so Wendell came back and kept him company. As they were going down a trail alongside the road where they had started, a sports car came up the hill at high-speed, downshifted with a great blast of exhaust and put Wendell's Arabian stallion into a bucking fit. He tried Fred's stunt of stepping off, but it was long off onto a hillside covered with head-sized boulders. He landed flat on his back. Wendell raised his head with some effort and muttered "Fred, would you please catch my horse," and then settled back on the boulders. Fred managed to catch the stallion and brought it back for Wendell to ride the rest of the way. Wendell's entire back was a mass of bruises, and his doctor pulled Wendell from competing that year, which was 1966.

At the beginning of the Tevis Cup ride the trainer brought Buck to the Lake Tahoe starting point and off went the riders in a gallop into the dark through thickets of small trees alongside the Truckee River and the highway to Squaw Valley. Several riders and horses ran their race before they even reached the starting point.

Gloria was Fred's assistant at the time and she met Fred and Buck at each veterinary checkpoint, along with the young couple from Fred's department who walked Buck around to cool him off while Fred did the same and ate and drank something before taking off again. Fred commented, "Buck never bucked again."

Wendell told Fred that he expected him to be the one to award the buckles later on Sunday at the banquet. Fred scribbled little notes about everyone in the ride. Either they passed him or he passed them where they chatted at the vet stops, which allowed him to say something about everyone. When it came Fred's turn, Wendell had arranged for one of their cohorts, the Director of the California Department of Forestry, to give Fred his buckle.

Wendell arranged for Fred to be the speaker at several lunch meetings of various riding organizations, which gave Wendell the publicity he wanted for his endurance ride.

Later Fred learned that one horse had slid off the trail during the ride and stumbled several hundred feet down into a canyon. The rider got off and was not injured. Wendell and some others went back down into the canyon to put the horse out of its misery. However, as they prepared to dispatch the poor thing, someone else showed up on the trail and it was determined the horse did not have any major injuries. Wendell paid $5000 of his own money to rent a flying crane helicopter to lift the horse out from the canyon.

Several years later, while working in Washington, DC, Fred saw Wendell on a trip to California. Wendell recalled that he had met Fred in

1934 when he had a trainload of snow brought to Berkeley in the San Francisco Bay Area to create a ski jump. Wendell had founded the Auburn Ski Club, and used this headlining stunt to promote skiing in the Sierra. Some 100,000 people gathered to watch as world-class skiers flew down the jump at 50-plus miles per hour. When Fred met Wendell on this trip, it was obvious that Wendell's mind had begun to fade, thinking that he had met Fred during the ski jump project, rather than on the trail.

Employees of Wendell's bank, Heart Federal Savings, said that Wendell often rode his horse to the bank and tied it up outside. He also always had a loaded 12-gauge shotgun on the wall behind his desk, which was situated next to Dru's desk. A couple of times a ruckus downstairs prompted him to charge down with his shotgun at the ready, able to dispatch the potential bank robbers, and creating quite a stir.

Fred heard another story about Wendell while he was participating in the filming of a commercial promoting his bank, Heart Federal Savings. Wendell, at age 84, played the role of "bullwhacker," dressed in his period-costume walking alongside an oxen-drawn Conestoga wagon, whip in hand. The wagon was moving along at speed, and somehow Wendell managed to fall along the trail, and the iron-covered wheels of the wagon ran over his chest and shoulders, resulting in fractured ribs, fractured collarbone and other injuries. Everyone thought he might be a goner, but he sat up and said, "When the front wheels ran over me, I thought, here comes the next son of a bitch," as the heavy rear wheels ran him over.

When Gloria (whom Fred had now married) and Fred purchased their lot in Auburn Lake Trails, they learned while on a short visit from Washington, DC, that the soil on their lot did not percolate, a requirement for sewage treatment. This was on a Friday prior to their departure on Sunday, and Fred wanted to get the problem resolved. So he called Wendell for assistance. Wendell contacted Georgetown Divide Public Utility District (GDPUD) and politely asked them to get a trencher down there the next day and find an immediate solution. A solution was found; the north side of their driveway actually did perk.

Wendell was obviously a man of immediacy. One of the local real estate agents told Fred he had a call from Wendell wanting to buy property, providing he could get the paperwork completed by the next day, which was somehow accomplished.

VII

Jim Steere, DVM:
Renaissance-Man and Athlete Extraordinaire
In Memory 3-15-1925 to 8-3-2010

When Jim Steere reached 35 years of age, he was in a midlife crisis. This crisis lasted for about 25 years. He was troubled, married, a doctor of veterinary medicine, and he had six children. He had just returned from Denmark on a Fulbright scholarship. It was the 1960s, and unbeknownst to him, other factors were to contribute to his existential questioning of how to make his life and career meaningful.

Living and studying abroad in Denmark made a significant impression on Jim. To illustrate, Denmark has zero population growth, complete medical coverage for citizens, and they view suicide as humane. Their values were certainly different than ours. One day, Jim, and a group of about 30 to 40 scholars took a bus tour of Hamlet's Castle. During the tour, there was a heated discussion about medicine, illness, and medical coverage. Jim remembered from that conversation that the Danes do not consider complete medical coverage as socialized medicine. In their country, a group of people hire their own doctor to treat their illnesses, and they called that practice a cooperative. If you were rich or employed, you would pay the doctor's fees. However, if you were poor or unable to financially contribute to the cooperative, you would receive government assistance to pay for the doctor's charges.

The discussion of suicide touched a personal nerve in Jim. In Denmark, suicide does not carry criminal charges, or have a religious connotation. Jim's grandfather, a California pioneer, committed suicide by ingesting strychnine. In the U.S., shame and guilt are associated with suicide, it's not openly discussed, and it's a crime and therefore punishable. The Danes are both more humanistic and progressive when it comes to depression and mental illness.

Jim had already invested money, time, and practical experience into becoming a veterinarian for large animals. He realized that he had lost his "God complex" somewhere along the way and that he was not going to become president of the United States. During this time, the major issues of the day included the Vietnam War, women's liberation, the pill, and the sexual and drug revolutions. Being young, intelligent, liberal, and full of endless energy, in the fall of 1963 Jim applied to Harvard, took the necessary classes, met the degree requirements and received a Masters of Arts in public health. After much soul searching, he decided to return to the Golden State to practice veterinary medicine, still unclear if his midlife crisis was resolved.

Several issues like growth, development, family, and environmental factors contributed to Jim Steere's unrest. Jim was born in 1925, on the fifth of March. As a two-year-old, his first memory was of living on the eastern shore of the Chesapeake in the state of Virginia. When he was three years of age his family moved to Berkeley, California. The youngest of four children, Jim had two older brothers and an older sister. Jim's father, Thomas Steere, is a story in and of himself. Thomas graduated from the University of California at Berkeley with a degree in engineering. Thomas became a commissioned officer in the United States Army without attending West Point, which was unheard of at that time. Thomas lived to age 96, and had a significant influence on Jim throughout his life.

Jim recalled vivid memories of early life as a child and adolescent, especially his father's behavior. He remembered being afraid of his father; his dad seemed angry much of the time, especially when he used foul language. On one occasion, Jim remembered his dad driving the family to Los Angeles in the Dodge touring sedan. Jim recalled his father yelling, "Goddamn that guy on my bumper!" and, "That stupid old bitch won't let me pass!" On that memorable trip it began to rain, and Jim remembered his dad allowing him to crank the wiper by hand, pleased that his father gave him that opportunity.

Jim's parents were married to each other three separate times. There were times in his life when he lived with both of them, and then with each parent separately. After his parents' first divorce, he recalled his mother saying, "I love your father and you should love him too. Your father loves us." Jim responded with, "Then why doesn't he come home and live with us?" Jim made his point. Receiving praise and validation was very important for him.

Another early memory for Jim was when Thomas moved to Virginia to teach at Greenbriar Military Academy. Florence and the children drove from California and camped along the way to visit their father. Even though Jim was a young boy, he already was an expert camper. Florence was not a typical parent or mother; she was ahead of her time. She earned both an undergraduate and graduate degree from Stanford University, with her master's degree in paleontology. She traveled alone to Berlin, Germany, to study sculpture. Florence lived to the age of 94.

When Jim was eight years old, he lost his older brother Charles. Jim believed that his brother's death had something to do with his parents marrying again. In that same year, the kids, Florence, and the Model-A Roadster traveled from California to the World's Fair in Chicago. Jim remembered how much fun he had riding in the rumble seat in that crowded car, stuffed with people, baggage, and camping gear. Some of Thomas's rants included, "Shut the goddamn doors," "Goddammit kid, you would forget your head if it wasn't screwed on your shoulders." During those scary moments, Jim wanted to stay away from his father as much as possible. Although his father never hit him, he threatened him with, "I'll tear your arm off and beat you to death with the bloody stump."

However, there were many positive aspects to Jim's relationship with his strict, verbally-abusive father. One time his father said, "Son, I'd like to take you on a camping trip to the Mojave Desert and show you where I lived for a couple of years when I was a boy." That particular trip was a birthday present for Jim, who was allowed to take along friends Brian and Theus. Thomas said, "We'll pack the Model-A and take off Friday a week from now. Step lively son; we have much to do to get ready for our bivouac."

On that particular Friday, Jim's father picked up the boys at the Los Feliz Grammar School. The group headed east into the San Fernando Valley, through Soledad Canyon and on to Antelope Valley. They came to the little town of Rosamond and then to Rosamond Dry Lake. To the south were the San Gabriel Mountains and to the north, the Tehachapi's. Thomas claimed that his father helped build the Southern Pacific Railroad. Jim's camping skills were sharpened as he learned more about nature's elements. Thomas taught him about the behavior of rattlesnakes, building a campfire, making roasting sticks with long tree branches and then sharpening the points to hold the hot dogs or marshmallows in place. Jim learned that prunes are good for the "constitution." He learned how to cook, wash the dishes, bury the garbage, and make the "poop pit." Jim received a first-hand education about living in the desert, which prepared him for the future. It was apparent that young Jim learned about affiliation, friendship, how to take in information and apply it as well. He also received valuable information about becoming a good citizen; being self-reliant, disciplined, and respectful of the environment; and the necessary components of a healthy lifestyle.

In 1862 President Abraham Lincoln passed the Homestead Act. "A homesteader has only to be the head of a household, at least 21, and he could claim 160 acres. He has to build a house, make improvements in the farm and live upon the land for five years in order to gain ownership." Jim's parents divorced again. His mom lived in Los Angeles, and his dad lived in the Mojave Desert on his 160 acres. Jim's dad wanted him to move to the desert and sweetened the offer by promising to buy Jim a horse that he could ride to school. Some would call it a bribe. Simply put, however, Jim wanted a horse and he liked the desert. He moved to the Mojave and united with his father. He helped his dad build a house, barn, and corral. They now had a one-room structure that contained a rock fire pit, a window and a door that faced east. They were without electricity, phone, gas, and water. One might consider that camping.

Good on his word, Thomas purchased a three-year-old bay mare, a Morgan. Thomas bought her for $100 at an auction—and this was during the Depression years. Jim named the mare Lady. Now they had to get Lady into the trailer to take her back to the ranch. After a lot of hollering and the stings of a whip, the horse finally loaded into the trailer and they eventually reached home. Thomas instructed Jim to give his new horse hay and water. "Let her eat, son," Thomas advised, "and get adjusted to her new home. First thing in the morning, I'll saddle her up and teach you to ride."

The next morning, an eager Jim and his father headed down to the barn after breakfast. His father took the halter and lead rope in his hand and they both entered the horse's corral. Lady saw them coming. Quickly, she laid her ears back, squealed, her eyes turned wild, and she charged, teeth bared. Jim was scared to death and ran toward the fence to get out of the corral. He noticed his father right behind him. So much for that riding lesson given by the great military officer! Jim asked, "What are we going to do, Dad?" to which Thomas replied, "Best delay for a while son, and let her settle in a little longer."

Jim was intelligent. After a while, he headed to the nearest pay phone in town. He called his mother collect, and was upset as he told her about the horse experience, especially his father, the Cavalry Officer's behavior. Florence calmed and reassured him, saying, "I'll be there this weekend I'll see what I can do." She added, "Make sure the mare has taken water, and be sure to talk to her every day over the fence. I'll see you Friday night, and don't worry."

Florence arrived on Friday and the next morning after breakfast, she walked to the corral to meet Lady. Florence was wearing pants, a rare occurrence. Florence calmly walked toward the unpredictable mare with a lead rope in hand. The anxious horse pinned back her ears and charged the new intruder. Jim's mother didn't move until the fast charging Lady was almost on top of her. And at the right moment, she somehow managed to wallop Lady across her nose. Lady stopped dead in her tracks. Then, when Lady's ears came forward, Jim's mother put a halter on her and laid the lead rope over her back. Lady finally began to relax, while Florence started rubbing her down gently with skillful hands. His mother then took the saddle blanket and rubbed the mare's neck and withers with it. She put the saddle on the mare and cinched the girth. Florence made an adjustment on the bridle, and placed the bit in the mare's mouth. Florence put her left foot in the stirrup, swung her leg over the horse's back and settled into the saddle, ready to ride. As he watched his mother ride off, Jim was utterly amazed. He couldn't believe what he saw. In that moment, his father, an officer in the U.S. Army Cavalry, seemed so inadequate.

When Florence returned she said to Jim, "Lady is very green. So I'm going to lead her with the lead rope while you ride on her back." Thus began Jim's riding lessons with his mother. "Horses are herd animals," said Florence, "and they get their orders from the herd boss. So when you work with horses and ride them, you have to be the herd boss and get their attention. When your father tried to work with her, Lady knew he was afraid of her and was not her boss. So she didn't trust him."

Jim never forgot that first lesson, which resulted in a significant amount of respect for his mother. What a marvelous lesson to learn. This lesson served him well throughout his life.

Florence spent a lot of time with Jim and Lady on that particular weekend and on weekends to come. Thus began Jim's attachment to his horse. He groomed her, fed her, and made sure she always had hay and water. When school started, Jim was eventually able to ride Lady to school by himself. At the beginning, though, Thomas drove the car alongside Jim and Lady as they trotted to school. Jim told his father, "You stop at the Texaco gas station and let me ride alone that last block to school. I don't want anyone to see my father riding shotgun for me in his car."

Jim was a fifth grader just beginning to master his equine and social skills, and a new way of life began for him as he bonded with his first horse. The horse was an important factor in his personal growth; it taught him responsibility, the importance of taking care of others, joy, independence, self-reliance, and self-esteem. His character and personality were nurtured at this young, tender age. Jim and the horse became one.

Jim spent the next five years on the windswept high desert. It was at least three miles to the nearest neighbor. In the winter the winds were fierce, and in the summer the winds were so hot that by noon, "I thought it was like being in Hell." Jim rode Lady during all the seasons to school and back, and together they herded cattle for a local rancher by the time Jim was 12. He explored overnight camping with his horse, and he could ride for 30 miles and not see a soul, a road, or even be stopped by a fence. While riding, he imagined himself as a lonesome cowboy or a prospector looking for gold. All these experiences helped Jim become excellent at nurturing his horse and taking care of himself.

Dinner capped off a typical day, following schoolwork and chores. After dinner, Thomas would light the pot-bellied kerosene lamp and Jim would make a fire in the fireplace. He sat close to his dad while Thomas read him stories about Tom Sawyer, Huckleberry Finn, and all the Penrod stories. Jim remembered one time when his dad told him he was going on a business trip to Las Vegas and that Jim would be ranch foreman until Friday afternoon when he returned. On that particular Friday, Jim came home from school ready to do chores, which included milking a goat named Lucy. But she was nowhere to be found. Then, he saw the dust of his father's car in the distance. Jim was afraid to tell his dad that Lucy was not milked. Jim got up early Saturday to look for her but couldn't find the goat. Lucy was still missing. Then Jim told his dad that he couldn't find Lucy that morning, which was partially true but also a lie of omission. Lucy was eventually found with a wound on her udder, torn skin flapping loose as she walked. Thomas told Jim to clean the wound and milk Lucy. He added, "I'm going to town to call the vet."

About half an hour later his father returned from town, followed by the veterinarian who drove a fairly new Chevrolet, and wore clean Levi's. The vet took one look at Lucy and said, "You city slickers." He took out his pocketknife, spit on it, and with a fast clean swipe sliced off the big flap of skin. He put some McKillop's Powder on the wound and told Thomas, "That'll be fifteen dollars, please." The year was 1937 and that was a lot of money—a week's wages for many folks. This experience could have been one of the reasons Jim became a veterinarian. Thomas wanted Jim to go to West Point and become an Army officer. But Jim didn't want to be anything like his dad.

Jim attended a schoolhouse with two rooms and a basement. His teacher from the fifth through the eighth grade was Ms. Burney, whom he thought was "terrific." Jim liked science and was good at it, and Ms. Burney got him interested in drama and music. According to Jim, she was the best teacher ever, bar none. He remembered the woodstove in the classroom that required a monitor to make sure it worked properly. If there was an argument between students, teacher Mr. Baer would take the kids into the basement, bring out the boxing gloves, and the kids would settle their differences right then and there. Jim definitely remembered the basement where he learned a little about boxing. He generally liked his classmates, got along well with them, and was, of course, the teacher's pet.

Jim's father decided that Jim should return to Los Angeles to finish junior high school. Jim asked his parents if they would allow him to ride Lady from the ranch to his mother's home in the Hollywood Hills 90 miles away. They both said yes, and Jim spent weeks planning the route. He needed to make sure Lady had new shoes, the tack was in good shape, and that both he and Lady had enough food for this long adventure. He also packed a sleeping bag and cooking utensils. His parents instructed him to call his mother in Los Angeles whenever he found a phone along the way. This was going to be a three-day horseback trek—his first three-day endurance ride.

By day one, Jim and Lady reached the foothills of the San Gabriel Mountains just short of Soledad Pass. On day two, they rode through Soledad Canyon past the little towns of Saugus and Newhall. The duo then reached the San Fernando Pass followed by the town of San Fernando. Eventually, Jim arrived at the Porter Ranch where the Porter family was expecting him. Lady spent the night in a box stall bedded with straw while Jim gratefully ate a home-cooked meal of meat, potatoes and milk.

Day three found Jim back on the trail with Lady, and by eight o'clock in the morning they headed toward the Hollywood Hills. They traveled through the towns of Pacoima and Sun Valley. In Burbank he crossed the Los Angeles River on his way to Griffith Park. Then it was a climb up 1800 feet to the top of Mt. Hollywood, and down to the planetarium to his home a half-a-mile away. When he arrived at his mom's house, his dad greeted him with, "Good ride, son, welcome home." Thomas shook Jim's hand, gave him a hug and said, "Son, I am proud of you."

During Jim's high school years, his parents divorced for the second time. Jim went to school in Los Angeles and spent his summers in the desert with his dad. In 1941, President Roosevelt called up the reserves. Thomas volunteered, but was turned down because of his age. He did, however, get a job at an Army airfield near Denver, Colorado. Thomas asked Jim to spend a year with him there. Jim told him that he would visit and then make up his mind about whether to stay or not. Meanwhile, Jim's girlfriend Diana moved to Illinois to live with her grandmother and Jim thought well, I'd be halfway there if I moved to Denver. So Jim hitchhiked to Denver, stayed with his father, and decided to attend high school there. As a senior, Jim was enrolled in Boulder High School where he made first-string guard on the football team and first trumpet in the concert orchestra. He sat next to the first French horn; a pretty girl also named Diana, and promptly fell in love with her.

Thomas went to every football game that senior year. One game in particular stood out in Jim's mind. The game was against South High, played on a cold and snowy night. The football was fumbled by a South High player, and instead of falling on it for a fumble recovery Jim reached down to pick it up. Unfortunately, there was a pileup and the opposing team recovered the ball. Jim was injured on the play, and was lying on the cold turf. His father leapt to his feet, ran onto the field, lifted Jim, and helped him off the field. The injury turned out to be a sprained knee, and Thomas nursed him by icing and massaging Jim's knee daily.

On December 7, 1941, Jim listened to the radio after church. He heard President Roosevelt asking Congress to declare war on the Empire of Japan. Jim remembered the president saying, "This day will live in infamy." Jim's father volunteered again and told the War Department that he was fluent in Tagalog, a Philippine dialect. Because of his age, 59, the War Department turned him down yet again.

Jim wanted to go home to Los Angeles for Christmas to be with the other members of his family. He rode in the car to Los Angeles with the superintendent of schools, who happened to be a graduate of Claremont. During the drive he told Jim all the good things about the school which directly influenced Jim applying to college at Claremont after he graduated from high school. In his first term at Claremont, Jim received a 'D' in English, history, and chemistry. He passed zoology and got A's in ROTC and gym (he excelled in football). He left Claremont and in 1943 was inducted into the U.S. Army Air Corps.

Jim wanted to be a hot-shot pilot, fly a P-38 and knock Japanese Zero fighter planes out of the sky. He spent 18 months in the Texas Air Corps and received his wings as a navigator and second lieutenant. His next base was at Victorville in California. There, he learned to be a bombardier and became skilled with the Norden bomb sight. Then he traveled to Boca Raton, Florida for radar training where he graduated as a radar operator, navigator, and bombardier. While Jim was home on leave, his paternal grandmother developed a serious illness. Meanwhile, his next assignment was to a B-29 crew at Grand Island, Nebraska. Jim asked for a compassionate leave to extend his time at home, which, lucky for him, was granted.

When he reported back to duty, he found out that his best friend, Bruce Seick, was assigned to his crew. For military purposes, the B-29's were stripped of all guns except those in the tail, which allowed them to fly high and fast. This elimination of guns enabled the plane to avoid the Japanese Zero fighter planes. So far so good. In April of 1945, Jim's crew flew from Grand Island, stopping in California to refuel, and on to Honolulu for a stopover. In the next leg of the trip they landed at Midway for refueling and then went on to their ultimate destination—Northwest Field, Guam. After parking the plane, the "Horny Hornet," Jim asked about his buddy Bruce. He was sadly told, "Sorry to tell you, Lieutenant. Bruce's plane lost an engine on takeoff with the full bomb load. It crashed and exploded on impact." Jim was in shock and realized that luck was with him. Jim's crew flew only one mission, and then the atom bombs were dropped—and just like that the war ended. They did, however, fly missions to the empire dropping food supplies by parachute to the prisoners of war camps. In Jim's group, there were 45 planes; nine were lost from flying accidents and none of the losses happened on combat missions.

In 1946 Jim returned to California and enrolled in Pomona College on the G.I. Bill, graduating in 1949. That year is extremely significant, because not only did Jim graduate; he also married Ardeth and enrolled in the new school of veterinary medicine at UC Davis in Northern California.

Jim graduated from veterinary school in 1953. He practiced veterinary medicine for five years in Oregon and for four years in Santa Barbara, California. During this time, Jim described his marriage to Ardeth as frail, and during that phase of his life he was hooked on amphetamines. He made it clear that even though his relationship with his wife was shaky at best, they both loved their children and were good parents. In 1968, Jim divorced Ardeth.

Sometime during 1968, Jim met a young, rich, and beautiful Mary Tiscornia. A torrid and passionate two-week affair resulted in a nine-year relationship. This relationship produced Jim's seventh child, daughter Jennifer who arrived in 1972. He knew it was almost impossible to live the life of a playboy and a veterinarian. He chose to be a veterinarian.

In 1967, Jim started his first Tevis endurance ride, but he wasn't successful. His horse was lame, and for the rest of the race he helped out by being a drag rider. By this time, he was a veterinary judge for NATRC competitive trail rides. Jim completed his first Tevis in 1968 and his last in the year 2005 at the age of 80, becoming the oldest rider to ever complete the Tevis.

In 1971, Mary saw an advertisement for a Ride & Tie competition event in St. Helena, California. At that time, neither Jim nor Mary were running and Jim had a smoking habit. He remembered the day in question as being very hot. His daughter Leslie came along as part of their pit crew to take care of her horse—a horse she loaned to Mary and her father so they could race. Up to that point in time, Jim didn't believe that two runners could literally run a horse into the ground. He remembered that there were 50 or so teams that included kids and Quarter Horses, as well as four teams of Buffalo soldiers. There was one vet check and the race distance was about 30 miles. At the vet check, Jim had his horse evaluated while his teammate Mary didn't stop but continued to run to get out in front of Jim and the horse. The horse's pulse did not come down at first, and the vet, an old-time cowboy veterinarian, said, "What is this hippie vet doing in this race?"

Jim became extremely angry, because when he took the horse's pulse it was about 65, but when the cowboy vet took the pulse, he said the horse had a pulse of 80, which meant the horse was not allowed to continue. Jim said, "I'll come back in five minutes." About five minutes later he returned. The vet checked the horse's pulse a second time. This time the horse's pulse and respiration now meet the vet's criteria so he was allowed to continue. Jim remained angry with that vet until the very end of his life.

Back on the trail, Jim came across a horse in trouble because of heat shock. He gently persuaded the rider to put the horse in the nearby creek to cool down. During this first race for Jim, two horses died from heat stroke and two other equines had problems as well. There was a newspaper article that reported about the horses' treatment (or mistreatment). Jim was quite disturbed about the newspaper article and what happened to those horses, and sought out a discussion with Bud Johns, the originator of the Ride & Tie. Subsequently, Jim became the head vet for Ride & Tie. It was clear that Jim was competitive and cared greatly about the horses, which says a ton about his character.

Jim wrote a letter to Bud Johns about how to help these competitive horses through proper vetting. Jim had educational, practical and experiential knowledge invaluable for the Ride & Tie sport. In 1972, Jim became the Ride & Tie head veterinarian, and his ideas about proper vetting to safeguard the horses were incorporated into the sport. Jim's footprint is clearly cast in steel in the Ride & Tie sport. It didn't hurt to have Peter Haas as one of Jim's clients, though. At that time Mr. Haas was one of the owners of Levi's. In 2008, Jim retired from being the head vet at the world Ride & Tie championship.

Jim acknowledged that he was competitive, liked to finish events, and had fun doing it. In his opinion, man is born to be competitive and it is part of our evolution to succeed. It certainly didn't hurt for Jim to have a mother who played women's basketball at Stanford in 1911. Having good genes, opportunity, and a nurturing environment all contribute to great opportunities for success, as we all know.

In 1977, Jim met D'ann at Indian Valley College where she was taking an animal health course from him. His story was that he kept mispronouncing her name. By the third week, he did it again. But this time an assertive voice replied, "That's D'ann, and don't you forget it." Then, according to Jim, he looked up to see who this person was and found himself gazing into the "most beautiful turquoise fire-filled eyes that I had ever seen." once again, Jim was in love.

Jim felt great. He no longer used drugs, nicotine or alcohol, and now exercised regularly. He believed this era to be one of the better times of his life, because he could still ride, compete, and was still in love with his wife. Looking back, he believed he tried too hard and did too many things. An example of that was when he was student body president at Pomona in 1948, where he met with the president of the college for one hour a week. He remembered him saying, "Jim, you have to watch your activities, and not let them get in the way of accomplishing things." He believed that it was very difficult for him to balance the necessary time constraints between work and family. He also believed, "If your mind and body are healthy, you can do a better job."

Jim thought that although the Tevis Trail was difficult, there were more difficult trails. The challenge of the Tevis was that you only had 24 hours to complete the ride. He remembered his last Tevis, at the age of 80, when a young man said to him, "How do you old farts do this?"

In 1977, Jim gave D'ann his gray Arabian mare Fatima. Jim knew that if Fatima had not been ridden for at least a week, she would buck a couple of times. After the mare bucked, she would settle down and be easy to ride. Jim, being the expert horseman that he was, told D'ann that he would first ride Fatima in order to get the buck out of her. Jim got on Fatima, and right away he felt her back begin to rise. She dropped her head, and "her haunches rose behind me." That was jump number one and he was still deep in the saddle. The second buck was a little higher and this time Jim's buttocks left the saddle. Jim thought he was in the clear. He wasn't. When she bucked again, Jim was coming down as she was going up and his crotch hit the pommel with the sound of pop. Jim was thrown and crashed, hitting the ground hard. At first he couldn't breathe, but when he was able to get his breath, he screamed, "Son of a bitch!" He then got up and felt his pelvis grinding. That short ride resulted in a hospital stay of two months with a diagnosis of a fractured pelvis and a ruptured bladder. After coming home from the hospital, Jim felt "totally committed" to D'ann and they set their marriage date for June.

During this time, Jim, D'ann, Florence, and Thomas were living in Thomas's Belvedere home. From April through May of 1978, Jim kept a journal of his father's health and ultimate decline. On the sixth of April Jim wrote, "Dad complained of hurting all over." On the eighth of April, Jim wanted to take his dad to Letterman Hospital. His dad replied, "There is no cure for old age, I won't live the month out. Keep me at home." On April 11th, he took his father to Letterman Hospital where Thomas received a diagnosis of pneumonia from Dr. Boyer. Even though they wanted to keep him in the hospital, Jim promised his dad that he would bring him home. On April 18th, his dad was bedridden, his eyes were closed most of the time, his body wasting away, and his speech was getting difficult to understand.

For the next 10 days, Jim watched his father's heartbeat rise through his thin chest. Jim described in detail the care, concern, and interaction with his dad, surrendering to the fact that his father was dying. Even though working at this time, Jim admitted "I hated to come home." Jim fed his father, bathed him, cleaned his bedsores, and massaged him. Jim described this passage as the "death watch." His father predicted that he would die by May first. Florence's birthday was the 13th of May, and Jim asked his father if he knew that her birthday was coming up. Thomas nodded in response.

Jim's dad was in great pain and needed relief, so Jim put in a call to Dr. Boyer. Thomas's therapy was Brompton's Solution—alcohol, morphine and codeine. By this time, the Marin hospice was involved. Jim told D'ann on May 9th, "I just had to get out of the room. The silence, then the raspy breathing, I can't take it any longer. The odor of dying, Lysol, urine, and the enveloping fog were too much. His wax-like skin pulled tight up to his skull, eyes slit open, sunken. And yet he lives on."

On the 10th of May, Jim wrote, "I would never let an animal suffer as my father has. I would have euthanized it days ago. Animals tell us when they have surrendered to death and are ready to die. How can I help you die, Dad? How can I help?" Jim added, "Dad, I'm here remembering all the good times and bad times we had on the ranch, gathering sagebrush, cooking on the wood stove, no electricity, hauling water, sitting on your lap while you read to me by the light of the pot-bellied kerosene lantern, riding my horse to school." His mother was cuddling Thomas in her arms, saying, "He's been a wonderful father and husband."

Jim began to reflect about how he might feel when his dad was no more. Jim wanted his father to die, because he couldn't take his own suffering nor his father's suffering. Jim wondered if he would be able to cry or if he was all cried out. Jim had a headache, but decided not to take aspirin or brandy. Then Jim began to reflect on his own death. "I will die as I've lived. Or, will I be fearful, anxious and afraid? Will I approach it as a new idea, adventure, or phase in my growing up? I believe, as I become oxygen deprived, I will see a kaleidoscope of lights, as I have in the past, when entering into that mystical space and disappearing into the vastness of the universe, from which I came."

May 13th was his mother's 88th birthday, and Jim wrote that his dad was quiet most of the day. After the party, Jim gave Thomas his Brompton's Solution, and his father said, "I'm dying. I'm dying. Help me. Oh, God help me. Jim, help me die. I love you, son. I love Laura. I love D'ann. I love Thom. I love Robert."

May 14th was Mother's Day. Jim woke up at 8:00 a.m., and he told D'ann that he was afraid to go into his father's room. From a distance he couldn't see any rising of his dad's chest.

Thomas was lying in Laura's arms, his face pale and yellow. Jim touched his forehead, and felt the warmth. But he realized that his father was dead. "Well dad, you carried out your plan. You made the party." Jim awakened his mother, announcing, "Mother, dad is gone." His mother replied, "Oh, I'm so thankful his suffering is over."

Jim's involvement with his parents demonstrated his love, empathy, caring nature and his humanness. It's clear that Jim Steere had a great capacity for love and nurturance for others. This was clearly defined at Jim's memorial service on August 22, 2010. D'ann, Robert, Thom, Becky, Leslie, Jennifer and the other kids were there along with hundreds of friends. Jim loved people and his friends loved him. Everyone at the service was teary-eyed. Although this man passed, he will never be forgotten.

Jim and I became close those last few years. I really got to know him much better while doing the research for this project. Prior to this time, I would call him with questions regarding my horse and ask about his well-being. He never hesitated to spend time with me, and always gave me the information that I needed. Even during one of my Ride & Tie events, I asked about lameness. Even then, he had time for me. I feel sad at this moment while telling this story. Jim, I love you. We all love you. You are missed. But you are part of us all.

Not to be forgotten, Jim at age 85, completed his last world Ride & Tie championship in June 2010.

VIII

22 Hours and 19 Minutes to Glory: Finishing the Tevis

My first endurance ride in the year 2000 was the Derby Ditch 50 in Nevada. The Nevada rides are not particularly scenic compared to the California events with their charming trails and vistas, nonetheless, I found myself camped in a fairly barren spot in Northern Nevada, getting ready to participate in Saturday's event. The plan was to camp next to the Shackelford family—Michael, his wife, and two children. Michael and 12-year-old daughter Rachel, both experienced endurance riders, were planning on competing and we decided to camp next to each other and ride together the next day.

The ride began along a trail that paralleled an irrigation ditch—the Derby Ditch. Not much stood out on this ride; it was neither exciting nor pretty. I do remember the last loop, however, which consisted of a long uphill climb. Our three horses were relatively close together as the finish line approached. Then, all of a sudden, we changed gait from a trot to a canter so we could race with a burst of speed to the finish. I was certainly pleased with how my horse Raider and I did. One ride down, two to go before the big one: The Tevis.

For the second endurance ride of the year, I drove to Redding, California, with trusty steed Raider in the trailer for the Whiskeytown 50-mile ride. I parked my rig next to Tom Christofk and Tony Brickel who were also competing. The Shackelfords were nearby. I remember clearly the rain that evening, and wondered how muddy the trail conditions would be. The weather, thank goodness, was fine for the race on Saturday. Riding in the rain is not my idea of fun. This ride had some tough hills with substantial elevation changes. Michael and I rode together, and of course we were some distance behind hot-shoes Tom and Tony. They always—and I mean always—ride fast in order to win. This day was no exception. I was riding for conditioning. I just wanted to finish.

Michael and I rode until we reached the last vet check. I was in front of him and stayed in that position until the last vet checkpoint, about 44 miles into the ride, where ultra runner Tom Johnson (three-time winner of the Western States Run) was assisting. I didn't realize that Tom Christofk and Tony were only a few minutes ahead of me; I used Tom and Tony as my yardstick for speed! Raider and I were in about fifth or sixth place at the time and I was surprised that Raider was that fast! Unfortunately, Raider clipped his rear hock and was sore. This resulted in us being pulled from the race which was a huge disappointment. There was one more endurance ride before the Tevis. My spirits were still high at that point, but I was in denial. With Raider pulled, it was unclear what that meant for the next race.

The next endurance ride was the NASTR 75, another Nevada ride. Tom suggested that Raider and I ride in the 75-mile division instead of the 50-mile ride. The 75 miles consisted of three long, hot, non-thrilling loops. The first loop seemed awfully long and the final loop was ridden in the dark. We had 18 hours to complete.

Once again, Raider and I arrived on Friday for a Saturday start. I specifically remember the start because Tom and Tony took off at a gallop for an early lead. Typical for those two; I was not surprised. Once again I wanted to just finish the ride. What I mostly remember about that day is how it was long and tiresome. I met two ladies on the trail and we rode together for hours. One lady was Barbara Johnson (no relation to Tom) and the other was Kelly Blue.

I finally finished the second loop, or I should say Raider and I did. Only one loop to go and then we were done, thank goodness. We came in ahead of Greg Kimler who is the owner of the Echo Valley feed store in Auburn and is a great sponsor of Ride & Tie. I was very happy to finish the ride successfully, and on top of that, beat Greg. Now Raider and I were ready for the Tevis, bring it on!

The Tevis is a logistical nightmare for rider and crew because of the long mileage and the geography of the trail. My official crew consisted of my friend Judy, her girlfriend, and Jerome Beauchamp. I was given a checklist by Debbie Brickel with information about crewing, supplies, driving instructions, and just about everything pertinent to the ride, at least from a crewing standpoint. Debbie, a three-time buckle winner, was so organized that by following her checklist, the whole process became much easier for my crew and me. She thought of everything, and I mean everything under the sun. At Robie Park (close to Truckee), the start line for Tevis, we were camped next to Tom Christofk, Tony Brickel, Michael Shackelford, and Becky Spencer, to name a few.

Because there were so many rigs and roads going in and around the campsite, it was difficult to find people—it's not like the campsites were lined up row upon row—people literally parked between trees where there were no roads. I had asked Judy to place a pie plate with directions about where we were camped near one entrance to the park so that Jerome could easily find us. Now, I probably don't need to tell you about how nervous I was, and how I was getting more and more uptight. I walked over to where the pie plate was tacked on a post, and found the pie plate turned around facing in the wrong direction. In other words, the information couldn't be seen from the route Jerome was arriving. My immediate emotional reaction was anger, but Jerome finally found us, with daughter Kaitlyn in tow.

After a long cooling-off period, I reached the rig where Judy, her friend, and Kaitlyn were all talking, laughing, and having a good time. My thoughts went something like this: "I better get some rest before the big day tomorrow and I only have a few hours to do that in." All right, there were more colorful words and phrases than I'm willing to admit to. I angrily asked the guests to leave the camper, but not before I got a bunch of flak from Judy. Finally, the guests left but I continued to be angry, and nervous. The ride start time was 5:00 a.m. on Saturday, which meant getting up around 3:00 a.m., a relatively short few hours after the incident.

I didn't sleep very well and the morning came exceedingly early. I groomed Raider in the dark, put on the saddle blanket, saddle, bridle and bit. I was ready to rock 'n roll! The plan was for Michael and me to ride together. Michael had started this ride but had never completed it. I had hoped this year would be different for him.

The beginning of this race was unlike anything else on the planet. There were now 259 anxious and spirited horses and scared riders in the dark, on a narrow road, waiting for the start. Everyone seemed so nervous and agitated. At the beginning of the ride, the trail was wide enough for a couple of horses to be side-by-side but then after a while much of it became single-track. In a single-track condition, it's extremely difficult to pass another rider because of the hazardous trail conditions. And at times, if you are in a group of horses, you are stuck until the trail widens. It's only then that you can safely pass. Otherwise it's like being in a parade.

I was not attempting to win this race; I just wanted to finish it. Michael and I got to Squaw Valley and both of us dismounted to let the horses drink in the nearby stream, where Michael and I had to be on opposite sides. There was not enough room for our horses to be together because of all the other thirsty horses. All of a sudden, Raider stepped on his reins and they broke. I was able to quickly make a knot in the reins and fashion them back together somewhat, but I didn't have a bit and I was without any control. Michael didn't see me and believed that I had left, so off he went. I didn't see him, so I left too. I wasn't very concerned about not having a bit to control Raider, because I often rode him without it while training. And during competitions, I would run alongside Raider, saving my horse's energy for later down the trail.

We were somewhere near Red Star Ridge, and the trail was extremely wet and sloppy from the snowpack. I was on the ground, attempting to get back on Raider when all of a sudden the saddle slipped to one side. I tried to hold my frisky horse still and tighten the cinch at the same time. Fortunately for me, Corey Soltau, a veterinarian from the San Francisco Bay Area, was passing on the trail. He stopped and grabbed my horse so that I could right the saddle and properly cinch Raider.

Raider and I arrived at Robinson Flat at about 11:00 a.m., having traveled around 36 miles, and finally saw Michael; unfortunately he had been pulled because his horse was lame. We talked about our earlier mishap and about our separation at the water hole. He knew that if he rode with me he would have a better chance of completing the ride. More than likely he went too fast. The trail was very technical and as the expression goes, "There's a rock out there with your horse's name on it."

For the next 20 miles or so, I rode with Matt Medeiros, an experienced Tevis rider and Ride & Tie competitor. Chris Turney, Tom Christofk, Becky Spencer, and Tony Brickel were all also out of the race, and these were all Ride & Tie competitors and experienced endurance riders.

After Robinson Flat, Raider and I were both feeling great and we continued to challenge the trail. After we passed the vet check at Last Chance and just before reaching Devil's Thumb, one of the riders blurted out, "We're in trouble because we're going to miss the cut off!"

I couldn't find my sheet with the cutoff times so I believed her and began to worry. If you didn't arrive at certain checkpoints within timing criteria, you got pulled. I was leading Raider up the many switchbacks, and then mounted him as we proceeded up to Devil's Thumb, thinking that this strategy would result in faster time. This climb had many, many switchbacks and was extremely steep. At this point, anxious about timing, I thought it would be better if I remained on Raider's back.

Soon after reaching Devil's Thumb (in fine time, I might add), I met another Ride & Tie competitor named Warren Hellman. It really helps one's soul to spend time with an interesting person, passing the time over long stretches on the trail, engaged in interesting conversations, and Warren fit that bill very nicely. Warren and I talked about a lot of things but what stands out in my mind 10 years later is a discussion we had about his early childhood and the circumstances surrounding how his mother passed. She had a brain hemorrhage while scuba diving and died while doing something she loved. What a great way to exit; by participating in a sport that brought you joy, camaraderie, and a few thrills along the way.

Raider and I, along with Warren and his horse Max, reached Foresthill at 19:58 after traveling 68 miles from the start. Foresthill is a vet check with a one-hour mandatory hold. Because of the dirt and dust, riders wore bandanas, looking like outlaws of the old west. I wore a painter's mask, the modern-day version of the bandana. Jerome, Judy and her friend met me there. Tony and Debbie were also there for technical assistance. They took Raider to the horse trailer so he could eat, and I followed along behind. I was hungry too. They took the saddle off Raider while I refilled my water bottles, restocked my power bars, and got everything ready to resume riding on down the trail. After roughly an hour, at 21:03, Raider and I left the vet check at Foresthill and again hooked up with Warren. It was beginning to get very dark and we were now mostly on the single track of the treacherous California Loop portion of the Tevis Trail. This was a difficult section of narrow trail because there was the mountain on one side, and steep, sharp fall-offs on the other side. If your horse took a wrong step or slipped, it spelled disaster for you both.

Luckily, horses have night vision, and the only way to compete in this ride is to maintain trust with your horse, including trusting that he can see what you can't. You don't want to flash a light on the trail since it interferes with your horse's night vision. If you trust your horse (and keep your fingers crossed) you are likely to have a safe journey, although certainly there are no guarantees.

Even though the ride took place on a full moon (called the "Comanche Moon;" it's the full moon with the longest time on the horizon during the year), it was still especially troublesome because of the cloud cover. This cloud cover made for a more difficult journey because of the absolute darkness. But Raider felt strong, and Warren and I wanted to make up time on this part of the trail. I was not afraid of the dark and was willing to risk the potential danger. A couple of times we found ourselves behind a group of riders going at a walk. We heard screams because some people were terrified of the trail and the dark. I still wanted to pass them. So finally, the riders pulled off to the side of the trail when they could, and we passed them at a good clip. This happened more than once, and we eventually passed a considerable number of fearful and timid riders. This part of the trail was approximately 20 miles of switchbacks, mostly downhill. What a relief to reach the next vet check—Francisco's. Now we had come 86 miles from the start. My goal was getting closer and closer.

After passing the vet check at Francisco's, we crossed the North Fork of the American River. There were lights and Glow sticks in and along the river so it looked as though you were walking down an airplane runway. The water was fairly high and reached my stirrups. Now, the aim was to get to the other side of the river, up on the bank, then off to the next vet check. Raider and I lived in this vicinity so we both knew where we were. After we crossed the river, as we approached Maine Bar (a trail we often took), Raider began to turn a hard left to go up this monstrous, ruddy, steep, long trail that took us to our warm and delightful home. It's as if he was saying, "I've had enough — let's go home." Normally, he's never thrilled to go up this difficult trail. But that night was different from all the other nights. I pulled his reins to the right so his head was aimed in the proper direction toward Auburn. I'm sure I said something akin to, "Remember, Raider, I'm in control. I am the rider and you are the horse." We continued down the trail that parallels the American River towards the Lower Quarry vet check, the last checkpoint prior to the finish. At this vet check we had completed about 94 miles.

Warren and I reached the Lower Quarry vet check at 01:59. Out of the vet check at a canter with a big grin on his face came riding none other than my friend Greg Kimler, who was riding fast toward the finish line so he could finally beat me. I wanted to get through this vet check as quickly as possible in hopes of turning this into a race.

Leaving the vet check, I got ahead of Warren because I was now on a mission. I wanted to catch Greg and finish in front of him. We crossed Highway 49 and then No Hands Bridge, trotting and cantering our way to the finish. Much of the final four miles at this point was uphill on a single-track trail. There were switchbacks on this portion of the trail, and we were in total darkness because of the dense tree cover. Raider caught up to Greg with about three other riders and horses. Raider and I somehow managed to get in front of Greg again on an endurance ride; however, this was no ordinary endurance ride. This was the big one—the granddaddy of all endurance rides—The Tevis. Of course, nowadays I remind Greg often of our ride in 2000.

At the finish line Raider and I were greeted by Tony Brickel. My crew was nowhere to be seen. It was 03:19 on Sunday at the Overlook near the Gold Country Fairgrounds. Raider and I took a victory lap around the track at McCann Stadium, and then proceeded to the vet check area. I was delighted as a kid in a candy store to be done with this ride. I was sore; mostly my back. I was thankful that Tony was there to trot Raider for the vet so the doctor could assess any possible lameness. Raider passed the examination, and then I was officially a Tevis buckle owner!

Tony led us to our trailer and I found Judy. We discussed the ride. She was tired and complained about how she didn't have any idea when I was going to arrive in Auburn, which was her defense about not being at the finish line. I was not sensitive, however, and told her that I bet my ex-wife would be jealous of me because I now had a Tevis buckle. My ex had talked about doing this ride for years. Needless to say, Judy was not thrilled with my sarcastic comment.

A few hours later, I led Raider out of his stall in anticipation of taking him home. But Raider had other ideas. He didn't want to get into the trailer. Luckily, Steve Shaw and Michelle Roush were walking by and I asked them for help. With their prodding Raider finally got into the trailer. Traveling from the fairgrounds in Auburn to Cool is about 10 miles so it didn't take long to get home. I put Raider in his stall area and got some rest myself before I headed back to Auburn for the awards banquet—and my buckle!

At the awards ceremony, I discovered that all my Ride & Tie friends had been classified as DNF, which translates to "Did Not Finish." Tom Christofk, Tony Brickel, Michael Shackelford, Becky Spencer, and Chris Turney were all part of that group. My friends were experienced, skilled, knowledgeable, and outstanding horse people. However, regardless of the circumstances, the completion rate for this ride was approximately 50% and had been ever since its inception in 1955.

The 2000 ride started with 259 horses and riders, and there were 126 finishers (49%).

At the awards ceremony, my name was called and I walked across the stage to receive my buckle. My friend Dale Lake (a Tevis completer, ride manager for 30 NATRC events and head of pulse and respiration teams for our Ride & Tie events) did hassle me by holding back the well-earned buckle. He then handed me my buckle, shook my hand and congratulated me; another goal completed.

This was my first major goal in a strictly riding event. I now had the prestigious Tevis buckle. Little did I know, I was not done with major goals in my life. After all, I was only 60 years of age. Thank goodness I was still passionate about running and Ride & Tie.

IX

2001: Significant for the Nation, Significant for Me

The year 2001 was both significant for our nation and for me personally. My mother was born in 1909, so she was 92 that year, living alone in Rockville, Maryland. One of her heart valves was replaced in the 1960s. And now, some 40 years later, she was having difficulty breathing, had a low energy level, and was very tired. She lived near my brother Ron, a physician, who was deeply involved in her medical treatment and care. Concerned about my mother's welfare, Ron had her admitted into the hospital in August. Ron, my sister Beverly and I, along with the cardiologist, decided that our mother should undergo a pacemaker procedure to help with her heart function.

After the operation she was in pain and miserable; the longer she was in the hospital the more she lost her will and desire to live. The longer she was in pain and discomfort, the more her health deteriorated. She just didn't get better in spite of this pacemaker procedure. Beverly and I realized we had pushed for this procedure because we selfishly wanted her to live forever. In hindsight, we didn't evaluate the situation properly nor did we think through the consequences of undergoing this procedure at her age. Sadly, her health became more and more compromised.

I visited mother in the hospital in September, staying with her until the 10th of that month before returning to California. We all know what happened on the next day, September 11, 2001. Of course, that day was a devastating shock that I'll never forget. I still remember watching the plane on television as it plunged into the World Trade Center, followed by tragic images of smoke, buildings collapsing, and people frantic. I could not believe what I saw.

The World Ride & Tie Championship that year was held in Euer Valley, California. But prior to this race there were a series of circumstances that played an important part in my life leading up to this event.

Judy and I spent November 2000 through February 2001 in Southern Florida. I was looking for a new horse when I received a videotape from Laura Christofk, an experienced and qualified horse person, whose judgment can be trusted without question. On the video was footage of a couple of horses for sale in Texas. After reviewing the video, I figured that on the way back to California, Judy and I could stop in Texas and look at some of those horses.

We left Florida and I had made arrangements to stop in Aubrey, Texas, to check out a bay mare. Unfortunately, Judy was distraught and depressed over leaving Florida and returning to California. Regardless, I made sure to visit this horse farm and meet the owner, Sherry. I rode Sherry's mare to evaluate her trot and canter. I liked the horse, but I wasn't in a position to make a purchase until I evaluated a few other horses. My friend Bob Edwards had a mare that I was interested in back home in California and I wanted to compare Bob's mare to Sherry's mare in order to make the best decision possible.

Once Judy and I returned to Cool, I made arrangements with Bob to bring his horse to my place so I could spend time with the mare. I rode her quite a bit and then asked my friend Kris Bartow, a veterinarian, to evaluate Bob's horse. He believed, along with my horseshoer Matt Mederios, that I could expect leg problems with this mare because of the horse's physiology. I listened to their input, and decided to not purchase Bob's horse.

Sometime in April, I received a call from Michael Shackelford, my endurance friend from Tevis. In addition to being an equestrian, Michael was also a pilot for American Airlines. He was looking for a gelding to purchase, and told me that Kris Bartow and he were flying to Texas on the weekend to look at some horses. He asked if I wanted to go along. "Yes!" was my immediate and enthusiastic reply, and so off we flew to Dallas, where we rented a car and headed out to find the perfect horse for each of us.

We visited a number of horse farms, and every horse we saw was first evaluated by Dr. Kris. He found something wrong with each and every one of those horses! I then told Kris and Michael about my earlier visit to Aubrey, and that I had seen a horse there that I was interested in seeing again. A chorus of three voices rang out with, "Let's go!"

I called home to get the phone number and then I rang Sherry. I got driving directions from her and off we drove to the ranch. Of the many horses we saw that day, that bay mare I had ridden previously looked the soundest. I made an offer on the mare, secured an appointment for a pre-purchase veterinary evaluation, and arranged to have her shipped to California if she passed the exam. As it turned out, I purchased this French Arabian mare and renamed her Gypsy Rose. She was my Ride & Tie steed for many years.

The next significant horse event for me was the World Ride & Tie championship. I didn't have a partner and young Gypsy wasn't conditioned properly for that race. I contacted race director Laura Christofk and asked her to help me find a partner with a horse. She referred me to Calvin Paulette from Washington State. I called Calvin and we agreed to partner.

Judy and I were having difficulties in our relationship. She was homesick for Florida and had a difficult time living in the country away from the city. I spent a lot of my time on the trails either running or conditioning my horse. Being a city girl, she didn't adjust well to my lifestyle. We parted and she returned to Florida

I drove to the championship by myself where I met Calvin. In the course of our ensuing conversation he told me that he had checked out the first part of the race, and suggested the following race strategy: I would start by riding the horse, ride until I reached the top of the mountain, and then tie the horse. Even though I had no firsthand knowledge of the climb, it sounded like a reasonable plan. I agreed.

The race commenced and I rode for quite a while, passing numerous horses tied to tree limbs. We climbed uphill—and more uphill—in what seemed like an endless amount of time. I began to worry about Calvin's ability to run that distance on this tough, long, steep uphill. I then did the unthinkable. I dismounted and tied the horse to a tree before I reached the top of the mountain. This was clearly not the race strategy that I agreed too. My clouded thinking led me to believe that I would help my partner by having the horse available sooner than what we had agreed upon so he wouldn't have to run that awful, difficult, uphill distance.

I eventually reached the top of the mountain, looking back periodically, expecting Calvin on the horse to catch me. He didn't.

After a while I knew we were in big trouble. I turned around and headed back on the trail looking for Calvin and his horse. There was no alternative at that point; this was the only logical tactic I could think of. I eventually found Calvin running up the trail, without the horse. I told him what I had done. He wasn't on the lookout for the horse, so he simply ran past the tied steed. I knew where the horse was tied (obviously) so I proceeded to run back down the trail to find him and ride him up the trail. Calvin continued running up the hill, so not only were we losing time, but now Calvin had to run more than originally planned. I screwed up, to put it politely.

Eventually, I found the horse right where I left him, and by now we were in last place. I rode and rode and finally caught Calvin. We did okay on that loop because I didn't make any more mistakes. We finished loop one, loop two, and then on to loop three. About halfway through loop three, a 12-mile loop, I found Calvin sprawled on the ground on all fours, throwing up on the side of the trail. He was done. He was finished. We still had another 4 to 6 miles to go in order to complete the race. The truth was clear, Calvin was barely alive and feeling horrible. I told him, "You ride and stay on the horse the rest of the way." I ran the remainder of the race and we eventually finished.

Major lesson: If you decide on a strategy before the race, stick to it. Make your adjustments by talking with your partner. It's a team sport. Both members of the team should be communicating clearly and understand the strategy. Another lesson is to not make assumptions about someone else's ability. Take care of yourself and be concerned about what you can and can't do. You can only control you. All in all, though, I was happy to have completed another championship.

My mother passed on September 24, 2001. This was a difficult time for me, and I didn't deal fully with her passing. I remember being sad, however, and having a miserable time at her funeral. Her body was shipped to Detroit and she was buried at Machpelah Cemetery next to my father. I said a few words at the service and remember crying like a baby while reading those meaningful expressions. It was an awful experience, and even now it brings tears and sadness. I still miss her and frequently have poignant memories of her. She was always there for me, regardless of my requests. I don't remember her ever saying "no." Her care, concern, and affection were unmistakable. Her support was unconditional.

I continued to feel guilty for pushing for my mother's heart operation. It's clear now that I wasn't thinking about her welfare. I wasn't thinking about the assault on her body, her emotional well-being, and the consequences of such an operation at her age. I hope never to make that mistake again. I got easily distracted and really didn't deal with my pain at that time; the emotions associated with loss were just too painful. Thankfully, a distraction quickly entered my life.

It was early October when I met three attractive women on the trail: Linda Rodgers, Judy Carnazzo, and Cindy Larkin. They were riding their horses near the 16-mile marker of the Western States Trail. I talked with Linda and she startled me with the question, "Why don't we run Western States in 2003?" I took that as a compliment! I replied with, "Let me think about it." That one question certainly made an impact. Linda was tall and thin with long dark hair. She was an extremely attractive woman with a bubbly personality. Who wouldn't want to train with her?

I began to research the Western States Run. Two of my running partners at the time, Joan Giniel and Audrey Viers, had both completed the run in years past. I called them and prodded and cajoled for information about this monumental event. I found out that if I was able to run a 50-mile event in under 10 hours, I could qualify for the 2002 Western States Run. Linda, because of her age (forty something), had to run 50 miles within nine and a half hours to qualify.

I also found out that the next 50-mile run, the "Helen Klein Race," was being held November 10th. So, I thought, why wait for 2003? Why not go for 2002? I called Linda and told her that we could enter the Helen Klein Race to help qualify for the WSER 100. Linda replied, "I'm running a marathon on that date." I told her to forget the marathon and go for the 50-mile race. She countered, "I've run a lot of marathons, but I've never run 50 miles." I smiled, "Neither have I! But I've run one marathon and one 50K."

I suggested to Linda that we do a 50K training run within the next week or so and that would prepare us. After all, after you've run a 50K, which is 31 miles, all you have to do is run 19 miles more! This is an example of my thinking. I employed denial on a consistent basis. After you've run 31 miles, what's 19 more? Obviously I've done an excellent job of repressing how I felt after my 50K. To top it off, I also forgot how I felt after I ran my first marathon. Oh well, Linda agreed. So we ran approximately 30 miles in early October. Then we both entered the Helen Klein 50.

I called Jerome Beauchamp and asked him to pace Linda and me at the beginning of the run. He agreed and joined us that Saturday morning. My running partner Joan also showed up. Linda (in her late 40s), Jerome (in his late 30s), and I at age 61 began the race together. We all had great energy that morning and Jerome ran with us for about five to ten miles. After Jerome left us, Linda and I ran together until I had to go to the bathroom. I never caught her again.

At about 25 miles, I became sick. Thank goodness Joan was there and diagnosed the problem: My Gatorade drink wasn't diluted enough. She threw my drink away and gave me some ginger to settle my stomach. We walked for a while and I soon began to feel better. Then I started running; I had close to 25 miles to go. My time for the first 25 miles was pretty good; about four to four and a half hours. Well, nothing dramatic happened for the next four to five hours, and I finished in about nine hours and 40-some minutes. I made it! Linda did well too and she beat the nine and a half hour time limit for her age group.

The Western States drawing for race entrants was held on a Saturday in December. It's essentially a lottery and 450 people are chosen. Linda went to the lottery. On that same day, Tom Christofk and Tony Brickel had a birthday celebration and a number of Ride & Tie people came out to run the Olmsted loop. I chose to participate in this run rather than attend the lottery, and then participate in the potluck hosted by Chris and Micki Turney. At about 11 o'clock, or so, I was in my vehicle after finishing the run, getting ready to leave when a smiling, joyous and thrilled Linda shrieked, "We got in! We're in the 2002 Western States Run!" I smiled blankly, unable to truly understand the impact of what she'd said, and mumbled something like, "Great, I'll meet you at Chris's house. Do you know where he lives? If not, follow me." If I had been thinking clearly, I would've said something like, "Oh shit!"

At the potluck we proudly announced, "We're in! We're in!" This was a running crowd, and attending this gathering were two people from Ride & Tie who completed the Western States Run some years ago: Chris Turney (two of three races) and Chuck Mather, who'd completed one time. Both men ran the race in under 24 hours. Chris was in his early 40s and Chuck in his early 50s. I talked with Chuck and asked him if he would be one of my pacers. He agreed. Now I had one pacer and was thinking about adding two more. As it turned out, Chuck paced me from Foresthill to the river crossing at Ruck-A-Chucky, and then across the American River to Green Gate.

From December 2001 to the end of June in 2002, I trained with Linda three to five days a week. Her husband Michael worked in the Bay Area and stayed there for most of the week. Her oldest daughter Amber was in college and her youngest daughter April in high school, so she had plenty of time to train. Linda was methodical, driven, and highly competitive. She printed out lots of training materials for this run, so I had written material about training and conditioning. And so began my education about ultra running.

The Epiphany, a 50-mile run, was scheduled for January of 2002 in the Oakland Hills and Linda suggested that we enter. Linda, another runner named Steve, and I showed up at the race site that Saturday morning. Only then did we find out that the run had been canceled. However, there was a man there who was in his running outfit. He knew the course and decided to do the up-and-back twice and use our car as an aid station. Essentially, the up-and-back was about 25 miles. No problem for the first 25 miles. The next turnaround was about 37-1/2 miles at Lake Chabot. Steve, Linda and the other runner reached the second turnaround before me and began to head back to where the cars were parked. I thought, "so far so good." Coming back, I made a wrong turn and got off course. I eventually got back on course, but became concerned because it was beginning to get dark and I didn't have a flashlight. Remember, the trail was not marked with the usual ribbons.

Linda knew I would be running in the dark and left a flashlight for me in a parking lot that we crossed on the trail, but unfortunately I didn't know that. When I got to the intersection where the trail, parking lot, and road met, I decided not to get back on the trail since I wouldn't be able to return to the car in daylight. I couldn't run in the dark, for the obvious reason that I couldn't see where I was going. Instead, I began walking on the road, hoping to hitch a ride back to my car. Eventually I was able to flag down a car. I explained my quandary to the driver, and he agreed to drive me to my car. When we arrived in the pitch black, Linda was extremely upset and worried. Going on the trail at night without light is a catastrophe, especially in January when the weather is cold and wet in the Bay Area. The decision to travel on the road and not the trail was smart. I lived to run again!

Linda and I ran every week until "The Run." We ran the Way Too Cool 50K and the American River 50 Mile Run. I ran the Jed Smith 50 mile run while Linda competed in a different 50 mile run the same weekend. During our runs together, we got to know each other exceptionally well and had a great bonding experience.

On Memorial Day, there was a three-day Western States training run on this rugged trail, which for many years served as the most direct route between the gold camps of California and the silver mines of Nevada. The trail's history echoed in my mind as I ran this route. The first day's run went from Robinson Flat to Foresthill (33 miles), the second day from Foresthill to White Oak Flat (20 miles), and the third day from Green Gate to Auburn (20 miles). Snow conditions caused a change in the start location for the first day. After the second day, Linda found out that her husband Michael had been injured in a horse accident and was in the hospital in Auburn. Later that evening, my then current girlfriend and I visited Michael in the hospital. He had broken a number of bones in his leg; he got caught in the stirrup while attempting to mount his horse.

After this three-day journey, my training and conditioning was essentially complete. I wasn't going to improve my performance by running hard or for long distances over the next three weeks. I had to taper off and be smart.

Weather conditions during the run were brutal, with temperatures roaring to triple digits in the canyons, contrasted by ice and snow conditions during the early part of the race. Elevation changes were extreme: From 6200 feet at the start at Squaw Valley, to 8700 feet at Escarpment, 6730 feet at Robinson Flat to 96.8 feet at Robie Point near the finish. This run climbed about 18,000 vertical feet and descended about 23,000 vertical feet from start to finish. Bears, cougars, and rattlesnakes lived in this territory. Every year there was a competitive field of world-class ultra runners, and this year's entries came from nine foreign countries, 42 states and the District of Columbia. This race was part of the Pacific Association's Ultra Grand Prix and was a big deal. On a fun note, we ran through the territory on the TV show 'Bonanza'. I planned to look for Ben, Hoss, Little Joe, and the oldest brother, whatever his name was.

I wondered if I was ready for my upcoming run. I completed two 5K runs, a half marathon, a marathon, two 50K runs, three 50-milers, and numerous Ride & Ties the last five years. My running resume was rather brief, to say the least. However, I hoped that my Ride & Tie experience was going to be my secret weapon and the key to my success. Up to this point, running competitions had been within ten hours. I had 30 hours to complete this 100-mile event.

During training months, I ran a lot and mentally prepared myself. I hosted a party for my three pacers: Jerome Beauchamp, Bill Johnson, and Chuck Mather. Chuck suggested that I consume at least one bottle of water per hour during the run to make sure I was properly hydrated. He was very knowledgeable about the California loop and agreed to pace me from Foresthill to Green Gate. That part of the trail was in the dark and extremely treacherous because of the steep 600-foot drop-offs. Bill Johnson, my second pacer, was going to meet me near Green Gate and stay with me until we reached the crossing at Highway 49. That part of the trail was in my backyard, so to speak. Jerome Beauchamp was to meet us at Highway 49 and take me to the finish line in Auburn. The plan was in order and complete. I liked my pacers and was feeling good at that point. It's funny how the mind works. At least I was confident about something; it might as well have been about my pacers.

While training for this major event, I made notes on the calendar. I recorded the number of miles that I covered, and kept track of the mileage on the two pairs of shoes that I used. Sometimes I recorded how I felt, or about the trail where I ran.

Steve Elliott suggested that I do a lot of standing to condition myself to the long time that I was going to be on my feet. Another friend, Dennis Burkett, advised me to take it easy the week of the run. He thought that I should go out for an easy jog or walk early in the morning for about an hour on Monday, Tuesday, Wednesday, and then rest. My sister Beverly, my then current girlfriend and I left for Squaw Valley on Friday, the day before the run.

Beverly arranged an interview for me with Susan Cohn Rockefeller, a friend of her personal trainer. This interview was going to be made into a film. I was interviewed before the run, during the run, and at the finish. The film was titled "Running Madness," which was obviously quite fitting.

There was a race meeting on Friday when outstanding ultra runners were introduced and first-time runners were asked to stand, at which time they received a standing ovation. That was a big deal and it felt great. Friday evening we met Linda and her mother and conversed about the Run. I brought my camper van and parked it at Squaw Valley, our home for that evening.

We all got up early Saturday morning. I ate, dressed, and checked in for the race. I placed myself near the front of the pack of 450 or so runners at the Squaw Valley start line. There was a rock-salt shotgun blast, and it all began. It was 5:00 a.m. Saturday morning. At this juncture, I was excited, adrenaline surging, and thrilled to be part of this exciting event. It was an awesome experience; the energy around me was phenomenal and the noise level was very high. I wasn't overwhelmed, but I was certainly caught up in the excitement.

We began climbing without the benefit of a chairlift as we proceeded up and over the Squaw Valley Mountain ski resort, site of the 1960 Winter Olympics. I remember walking and when the mountain trail leveled off, I started running. I recall the snow on the ground and all the nasty, hungry mosquitoes. I did not prepare for that. When the sun rose, runners began to drop their outer layers literally on the trail. There was an enormous amount of nervous energy that morning, swirled together with a lot of chatter. I remembered to drink and eat as I proceeded with this massive herd of runners.

I reached the first checkpoint at Red Star Ridge some 17 miles into the Run. Acquaintance Leigh Bacca made an offhanded remark, doubting my ability to get that far. Friend Chuck Gabri grabbed my arm (in a friendly way) to hold me steady, which actually felt good. Chuck was the aid station captain and has completed both the Tevis (six times) and the Western States Run. Later I found out that he had bet that I would not be able to complete the run. Up to that point there was no support from crew; they were simply not allowed on this section of the trail.

I remember arriving at Robinson Flat about 30 miles into the run and meeting my crew. My choice for sustenance was a turkey sandwich, electrolyte tablets, and Gatorade. The film team took a shot of me as I yelled to them (undoubtedly something profound). Beverly encouraged me while she walked with me a short way.

I made it a point to move quickly through the aid stations, because I was concerned about making the time cutoffs. The temperature was rising, and I was conscious of the need to consume water and electrolytes. I got ice from my crew and put it under my cap to cool my body's core temperature. I was literally focusing on keeping one foot in front of the other. Runners were more and more spread out; when we did come together we chit-chatted with each other. There were periods of alone time, and my mind wandered. I thought about when I grew up, and I thought about the miles I had completed. This process helped me continue on. I was tired.

At the next aid station, about five miles in, I was happy to see my friend Kellie Holsey working. I don't remember much other than running, walking, eating and drinking for the next 25 miles or so. I went up Devil's Thumb, 40-plus miles into the run. It was comprised of about 50 switchbacks from the river to the top of the climb that seemed to go up to the sky. This was much harder than the Tevis. And, I might add, the name Devil's Thumb is appropriate. Along the side of the trail there were runners sitting, puking, and looking like dead men and women. We were now in the canyons; it was hot, getting hotter, and I was exhausted. It took grit to continue. Thank God I got through that part of the run without any incident.

At the 55-mile marker, I reached Michigan Bluff. This little community was the first sign of civilization. I saw Matt Medeiros leaning over the balcony of his house, which was adjacent to the trail. He said, "You didn't think you'd get this far, did you?" That remark pissed me off but was good motivation.

It was now about 7:30 in the evening, and my crew was at Michigan Bluff, thank goodness. Judy Carnazzo helped me change into a clean shirt. It felt good to get rid of my dirty, sweaty one. The weather was now becoming my friend. It was starting to get cooler, compared to the triple digits up to this time, and I was more familiar with this part of the trail. At each stream crossing I took my cap and wet it to cool myself down.

It was on to Foresthill, 62 miles into the run, where I met my crew and pacer Chuck Mather. I was extremely exhausted at this point, to put it mildly. I told Chuck he could talk to me, but not to expect a reply. I didn't want to talk; I simply wanted to save energy. He fed me GU constantly. He also helped by holding onto my shirt while going downhill in order to keep me in an upright position.

When we reached the deep American River crossing at Ruck-A-Chucky at 78 miles, I had to step on the scale to check my weight. Let me explain. Periodically, there were mandatory weigh-ins along the trail, and your weight was recorded at the beginning of the run. If a runner was to sustain a weight gain of over 10 to 15 pounds, he or she would be automatically pulled. If you were gaining weight, your kidneys had probably shut down. Anyway, Chuck pushed me up to the scale and held me while I got on. My quads were shot, which meant I couldn't run the down-hills anymore. I had to traverse them slowly. However, my kidneys were working.

Then we proceeded to the river crossing. There was a cable going across the river to help the runners and pacers steady themselves. The object was to hold onto the cable and not be swept away. The water rose to my waist; it was cold, coupled with a fast-flowing current. The river rocks and boulders were extremely slippery and sharp. We eventually reached the bank on the other side. I was now closer to finishing this grueling event. A three mile climb to the Green Gate aid station was the next goal. It was easier to go up hill than down because my quads hurt. My other crew, Bob Edwards and Jim Harris, were supposed to meet me at Green Gate and bring me another pair of shoes, in addition to food and drink. My body had begun to shut down and I had lost my appetite back at the California Loop, quite a few miles ago.

My buddies were not there when Chuck and I arrived at Green Gate. I didn't wait for them. Chuck Mather finished his job of pacing me to this point and left me in the capable hands of Bill Johnson, my second pacer. Bill and I proceeded in the direction of the next aid station at Auburn Lake Trails. Bill attempted to motivate me to run faster by telling me, "Linda's just ahead of you." During this part of the run, Bill fed me countless Fig Newton cookies, the only thing I could eat. It was now early morning when we reached the old campground just below my house and 84 miles into the run.

My friends Fred and Gloria Jones were there waiting for me. Before the run, I asked Fred to bring me a Popsicle at this aid station. Fred, being the scientist that he was, tracked me on the computer, and knew exactly when to deliver the Popsicle that was kept cold by being packed in dry ice. Perfect! I had my Popsicle.

Approaching the next aid station, Brown's Bar, loud rock music could be heard wafting in the air. The aid station volunteers were dressed in silly costumes, and the atmosphere was completely party-like. This was the best aid station ever. I only had 10 miles to go, and the celebration was appropriate. Bill and I continued to the Highway 49 Crossing. I had now completed around 93-1/2 miles. It was still not fun, but I was making progress.

Jerome Beauchamp was waiting to take me the rest of the way to the finish. I saw my crew again at No Hands Bridge. They were wonderfully ebullient with more special encouragement. I had only four miles to go and Jerome encouraged me to pick up the pace, pick off the runners, and get ahead. His approach was just what I needed; in fact, it was splendid. This prompting gave me something to think about besides how tired I was. I liked the feeling I got when I passed other runners. It was a great motivational tool.

Now I was at Robie Point, the top of the climb. I was met there by Tony and Deb Brickel, Bob Edwards, Beverly, and Marissa. Bob wanted me to run faster. I wasn't going to listen to Bob, and chose to stroll. The remaining mile-and-a-half was along the streets of Auburn and I was feeling surprisingly good at that point.

Then we arrived at the high school track, where all that was left of the Run was a quarter of a mile to the official finish line. At this 'victory lap' I started running fast since I had good energy. As I crossed the finish, my name was announced and I saw my time overhead. There was a lot of noise from the much-appreciated friends, runners, crew members, pacers and public in the bleachers. I completed the 100.2 mile run in 29 hours, 13 minutes, 06 seconds. What a relief! I was pleased, to put it mildly.

I was now ready to collapse and a wave of tiredness overcame me. I was interviewed again for the "Running Madness" film and then we left for home. Once I got home, I puked on my lawn and simply lay on the welcome and delightful bed inside. My quads and hamstrings were shot. In all honesty, they were actually torched by the time I reached Foresthill. Thank goodness for my pacers. I could not climb the stairs at home, let alone get down them. Luckily, I had a bedroom on the first floor. A couple of hours later, we got back in the vehicle and returned to Auburn for the awards ceremony.

Back in Auburn, I met up with a bubbly and joyous Linda, who had also finished. We stood in line to receive our buckles. If you finish within 24 hours, your buckle is silver. If you finish within 30 hours, your buckle is bronze. I received my bronze buckle. And then, presenter Greg Soderlund said something that I didn't comprehend. Greg reached behind the awards table, whipped out a box, and awarded me with a jacket commemorating the fact that I was an age division winner in the 60-69 grouping. This was a total surprise! Not only did I complete the run, I was also a winner in my age division. I was extremely proud of that.

I still feel proud of myself for doing that run. It's an example of training, hard work, determination, mental toughness, and putting one foot in front of the other. I remember telling myself during the difficult times, "I can." Saying that certainly helped me get through the run. During the night, between Foresthill and the river crossing there were numerous runners sitting alongside the trail. Chuck always kindly asked them if they were okay. These memories remain. I have pushed away some of the memories of the more difficult periods during this 29 hour undergoing. But I continue to wear my Western States Run jacket and belt buckle with great pride and honor.

In the 2002 Run, 255 participants (of the 450-plus who started) were awarded finishing buckles. Statistics for that run suggested that there was about a 50% completion rate, even with the strict participation criteria. Over the years, Ride & Tie individuals have done very well in this race. For example, Jim Howard had two victories and Tom Johnson had three victories and held the course record for the 30-39 age group, Brian Purcell had one victory, and Mark Richtman came in third in 2002.

I found out later that only 40 individuals, or so, had completed both the Western States Run and the Tevis Cup. Gordon Palmer completed the Western States Run in 1983 when he was 44 years of age; he also had 11 Tevis buckles. He told me about Gordy Ainsley, two-time Tevis finisher (1971, 1972) and the first man to complete this run. In 1974, according to Palmer, 27-year-old Ainsley was trying to borrow a horse for the Tevis, however, no one would lend him a mount. Apparently he rode heavy in the saddle, which made it difficult for the horse. He asked Dru Barner (Wendell Robie's secretary) if she would loan him a horse. She said, "No." Wendell suggested to Ainsley, "Why don't you run it alongside the Tevis horses?" Dr. Lind, part of the Tevis management said, "No man can do this in 24 hours." Wendell Robie bet him that Ainsley could.

In 1974, Ainsley found himself in the midst of clouds of dust and the ring of hoofbeats as he ran alongside the horses during the Tevis Cup Ride. Gordon Palmer was there, helping out as crew. He remembered filling empty soap bottles with water for Ainsley to take with him to the next vet check. Palmer wasn't sure that Ainsley could do it in part because there is so much dust on the trail, making it difficult to breathe. Ainsley finished that run within 24 hours with about 17 minutes to spare. He would have been faster but he spent time helping a rider with her horse. Incidentally, Ainsley competed in the second world Ride & Tie championship in 1972 and came in fifth with his partner. In 1973 he came in second and in 1974 came in first with his partner Jim Larimer.

So, Wendell won his bet. Man can complete this 100-mile adventure on foot within 24 hours.

In 1976, Ken "Cowman" Shirk completed the run in 24 hours and 30 minutes (alongside the horses), and he finished the Tevis in 1982 and 1983. In 1977 Cowman completed his first world championship Ride & Tie.

In 1977, the Western States Endurance Run became official. In

1979, Wendell decided he didn't want the Tevis to be associated with the run. More and more runners entered the event. Runners were happy not to have to deal with all the dust from horses. In 1981, the run separated from the ride and incorporated a 30-hour time limit.

My friend Chris Turney, an outstanding collegiate runner, and a 24-hour Western states runner in 1986 and 1988, talked about all the peaks and valleys that the runner goes through during the event. For him, during his lows it seemed everything was hurting—his feet, his stomach, and there was the constant feeling of nausea. He began to question himself: "What did I do wrong?" "Did I drink enough?" "Did I do enough heat training?" He had plenty of self-doubt. Eventually, Chris was able to climb out of his despair. His adrenaline flowed and he got the infamous "runner's high." He felt better and began to run faster. While running like the comet Mercury, he noticed the pain on the faces of the other runners. He felt sorry for them and was certainly empathetic, but he also experienced pleasure, a sadistic quality that made him glad it was them and not him. When he was feeling good, it was only then that he could enjoy the beauty of nature that engulfed him. Chris understood how the longevity, length, and frequency of all the climbs and the accompanying descents resulted in havoc on one's muscles. Fatigue and muscle breakdown take over. There was excessive lactic acid, muscle soreness and exhaustion to be dealt with. It is not uncommon to see other runners limping, hobbling, bent over, and crooked. At times, it's like being on a death march, the kind you see in the movies. Pain and agony are part of this run. We do it voluntarily. The question "why" comes to mind and we continue to ask that question.

X

"Dr. Ironman" Lew Hollander

Lew Hollander, born June 6, 1930, is 5'10" tall and weighs about 180 pounds. This 80-plus year old male has completed 21 out of 21 Ironman competitions on the big island of Hawaii. The Hawaiian Ironman went well for Lew in 2009 for his 20th completion. There was a considerable headwind but his finishing time was 16 hours and 54 minutes. His 21st race completion at 15 hours and 47 minutes in 2010 made him the second oldest Ironman finisher. Incidentally, his finishing time in 1985, his first Ironman, was 15:48. A mere one second difference in a span of 25 years! Lew excelled in running, biking, swimming, tennis, ping-pong, Ride & Tie, and endurance riding. However, his athletic prowess was only part of the story. In addition to being an author, Lew described himself as a scientist, with a career in physics that spanned from atomic weapons testing to semiconductor research.

Lew claimed that as far as triathlons go, swimming was his strongest segment. His biking ability had greatly improved over the years, and he stated that as far as running goes, he could run "forever." At that point in time, he did not consider himself fast, but steady. Lew believed he was blessed with fast-twitch muscles and thus was able to recharge quickly. An example of the phenomena was when he finished a marathon, he could still run and continue to run and run because he was not overly tired. His fast-twitch muscles were important factors in his running success. He could run sprints and was also successful running at longer distances. When Lew was running in competition, he ran his own race and did not get caught up in what the other participants were doing. He didn't run by the clock or by what others did, and kept within his own abilities. He used the latest high-tech equipment, owned a state-of-the-art bike, and wore a fast-design swimsuit for competition.

In 1984, Lew completed the 100-mile Western States Run. He did it once, commenting, "That's enough." He completed every running race he entered, which speaks to his mental and physical toughness. After conquering the Western States Run, he wanted a new challenge and began looking for another sports activity. He thought about triathlons but didn't have a bike at the time, so he simply purchased the best bike money could buy. A major consideration in triathlons or Ironman competitions is the ability to transition from long-distance biking to long distance running. Different major muscle groups are used for each sport.

Lew knew that he could easily make the transition from biking to running, reasoning that his Ride & Tie experience would be a solid gauge. As an excellent competitor in Ride & Tie, Lew thought that making that transition in triathlons would go well, and it did. When he started bike training, he found that he could then transition to running. Now, all he had to do was increase and build up the many miles needed in order to handle the biking part of the event.

Lew was an excellent swimmer. Jokingly, he said, "I'm not going to drown because I'm not afraid of the water. (In the Ironman) I would be doing the same things I did as a kid—swimming, running, and biking, but now I can do them better." Lew was healthy and hoped to remain so as long as possible. He attempted to keep within the limits of his abilities as his mind and body worked in harmony and as a consequence to his maximum potential. He figured that today he was running well, but not necessarily faster than in the past. He got tired after competitions, and realized his recovery time was not as fast as it used to be. He now rested for longer periods of time after competitions. He had planned to skip the Ride & Tie event because he always wanted to do his best in every event that he entered, and he feared that he might not recover sufficiently from the Ironman the week before. In years past, he would have done both events without question and not concerned himself with the issue of recovery time. Lew was a thinking man; he planned ahead, was aware of his limitations and attempted not to compromise his physical abilities.

However, things changed and Lew completed the world Ride & Tie championship in 2010, and was awarded with being the oldest finisher in the long course.

He continually asked himself, "Did you do the best you can, Lew?" That was his philosophy in a nutshell. He liked the challenge and the prestige of doing well.

Lew often talked about two other Ironman competitions. One was in Japan; at the age of 65 Lew was the oldest winner. He remembered, "They clapped for 10 minutes. I was a hero! They were impressed, which reflects their cultural respect for the old." The other one occurred in Germany when he was a youthful 70. Recognition is such a great reward for accomplishments!

In 2009, Lew completed several half triathlons and qualified for the big one at Kona, Hawaii by winning at St. Croix. His planning and looking to the future were important components to his success. Also important was the difficult training he put in during a 24-hour day. But if you ask him, he might refer to training as just playing . . .

When Lew was about nine years old, he experimented with mixtures of chemicals that would explode, ". . . and explode they did," smiles Lew. "I have always wanted to be a scientist, for as long as I can remember, even though my mother did not think a person immersed in physics could make a living other than by teaching."

As a boy, Lew was very pleased with himself as long as he could make a bomb and make it go bang. He wrote his first scientific paper when he was nine. Lew realized at a very young age that our society rewards those who can make a bigger and better bomb. He sent a letter to the War Department describing his technique in mixing certain chemicals and the ability to set off an explosion. The government sent a letter back, thanking him for his contribution, adding, "We want it to go off when we want to."

Lew had competed in sports for a long time. In Long Island, New York, where he played high school football and baseball, Lew graduated at age 16 because he skipped two grade levels. He received his bachelor's degree from Adelphi.

One disappointment occurred early in his life when Lew played running back in high school, and believed he could do the same in college, so he went out for the football team. He claimed he got banged and beat up during football practices, and to his surprise and disappointment, he didn't make the football team.

After graduating from college Lew enlisted in the United States Navy. Following his time in the service, he enrolled in graduate school and earned a Ph.D. from Lincoln. His area of expertise was (and is) solid-state physics.

Lew took a series of tests in the Navy. Scoring the highest in a group of 200, Lew was fast-tracked along and became a commissioned officer at 21 years of age. This young man was assigned to the U.S. Naval Radiology Defense Laboratory in San Francisco, California, commenting, "I had the best gig in the military." In the Naval laboratory, he was introduced to Nobel Prize winners, scientists, and professors from the most prestigious universities. Fortunately, he was given the opportunity to work in each of the various divisions in the laboratory and was able to pick the division he liked. Not only that, he played shortstop for their baseball team and was the only officer in the lineup. He acknowledged that he really didn't have a strong arm and his natural position was playing second base. However, being an officer, he was the shortstop.

Lew had many accomplishments during his time at the lab. For one, he wound up building the world's best X-ray machine that calibrated radiation. He also developed crystals that measured radiation, and at the age of 22 Lew developed scientific instruments like the radiation sensor. Upon leaving the service in 1955, he was told by the Navy that they would give him a contract to build his device regardless of the company he chose to work for. Not bad for a young scientist. Over the years Lew wrote and presented scores of scientific papers and developed numerous patents. At age 80, he continued to present papers at scientific meetings and was granted patents for his various inventions.

Some may ask whether he used his scientific background for anything else. What about applying scientific ideas to endurance riding?

Lew is a member of the American Endurance Ride Conference (AERC) Hall of Fame, and has ridden nearly 11,000 endurance and Ride & Tie miles. He has over 150 wins and best condition awards. Best condition awards are coveted; in fact, many riders would rather have the best condition award than come in first in a 50-mile or 100-mile endurance ride. Lew has also competed in over 21 world championship Ride & Tie events.

If you want to learn more about endurance riding, a good source is Lew's book, "Endurance Riding, From Beginning to Winning." This pioneer introduced numerous ideas, techniques, how-to tips, and standards that are now part of the sport today. In Lew's book, his focus is introductory information that helps new riders in the sport of endurance riding. Additional information includes scientifically-developed strategies to help the rider obtain the best possible performance from a healthy and sound horse. Lew also included a chapter on Ride & Tie crewing; this book is a tremendous resource for the Ride & Tie and endurance participant.

To illustrate Lew's idea of successfully passing a vet check at an endurance ride, the following is extremely informative: It's important to get through the vet check as quickly as possible. The rider does that by making sure his horse has met the pulse and respiration criteria before entering the vet check area. One way to do this would be to dismount from your horse prior to entering the vet check area. In addition to dismounting, the rider loosens the saddle girth to assist the horse by helping him to relax and breathe more easily. The rider can also walk or trot alongside the horse on the way to the vet check to allow him to catch his breath. Upon reaching the vet check, the rider can immediately call a volunteer over to get the pulse and respiration (P&R) readings on the horse. If the horse has met the established P&R criteria, then the hold time begins. This is good advice and exactly what the rider should do, because the sooner the horse has met the criteria the quicker the rider can continue the race.

This procedure of the 'hold' beginning when the horse has met criteria was introduced by Lew at an AERC convention a number of years ago and is now called the "Gate to Hold." This man also coined the AERC slogan, "To finish is to win," and developed a recognition program to award rider mileage.

Of course, the underlying motive in all this is to make sure the individual takes care of their horse properly. After equine electrolytes became popular for use on endurance rides, Lew came up with his own brand of inexpensive and available mixtures of various types of salt which he called Lew's Mix. It may not have been a bomb, but apparently Lew still mixed things together well! He also developed a usable high-fat diet for horses.

It's also important to note that Lew's wife of 43 years, Hanne, was also an endurance rider and was also inducted into the AERC Hall of Fame.

It's easy to understand how Lew became involved with endurance riding since he's had horses for most of his life. A legend by the name of Julie Suhr (the first person to ever achieve 20 Tevis buckles and author of "Ten Feet Tall, Still") introduced Hanne to endurance riding. Julie and Hanne rode together, and it was Julie who encouraged her to start endurance riding. Hanne started her endurance career and according to Lew, she was happiest when she was riding. According to Hanne, her life is defined by, "Born to ride, forced to cook."

Early on, Lew wanted to do endurance riding but he didn't have a conditioned horse. He did the next best thing—he borrowed one from Pat Browning. In all likelihood, if it wasn't for Julie, Hanne, and Pat Browning, Lew might not have competed in endurance and Ride & Tie.

Pat Browning and Lew first met in 1972 at the Castle Rock endurance ride hosted by Lud and Barbara McCrary. Lew volunteered to monitor a cattle guard crossing. His job was to make sure that the horse and rider did not step on a cattle guard grate (a horse could easily get its foot stuck) but went around it instead. Pat and his horse actually jumped the cattle guard! That's when they first met. After that ride, Pat put on his own endurance ride called the Nugget 50. Lew arrived at the Nugget with a lame horse, so Pat gave him one of his horses to ride. According to Pat, "Lew is one of the toughest men ever. He doesn't look like it, but he is a brain." Pat added, "I had to work like hell to beat him in all our competitions."

Dick Guelich, Lew's good friend and business partner for 50 years, was instrumental in finding a wife for Lew. Dick wasn't happy with Lew's dating choices and realized that Lew was not at his best in the work world and was, in fact, troubled by the lack of a solid relationship. Dick suggested that Lew go to Denmark and find a Danish farmer's daughter. Dick then bought an airline ticket for Lew to go around the world. Dick put him on a plane and Lew flew off to Denmark.

Upon arrival, Lew went to a dinner club where you could dance, eat good food and meet pretty girls. Hanne arrived at the club with four other attractive girls. She wore glasses and had a great smile. Not being bashful, Lew went over to her and asked, "Would you like to dance?" It was no accident that she grew up around horses. Lew wound up staying a month in Denmark and that was 43 years ago. Needless to say, his unhappiness and imbalance were erased. Hanne had a tremendous influence on Lew and played a significant role in his successes in endurance riding, Ride & Tie, Western States, and triathlons.

One day Lew and Hanne were riding in one of the national championship rides, a total distance of 200 miles. This was an important race because his wife would be the likely winner. The trail was steep and rocky and it was during the night. They were in first place at that point and they could see a light in the distance which was probably the next closest rider. As competitors, they did what was necessary; they both galloped their horses downhill in the dark until they reached the flat part of the trail. Lew asked his wife, "How could you ride that way?" Hanne replied, "We ride that way all the time." He countered, "Yes, but during the daytime." Hanne replied, "I can't see the trail in the daylight." This was a good example of being able to trust your horse. Thank goodness the horse had good night vision, as the ride must go on. Here was another example of being goal directed, aggressive, and having mental and physical toughness.

Being aggressive and being able to control one's aggressiveness are important characteristics of the successful athlete. Lew's aggressiveness was evident at a very young age, and although he has been able to sublimate it in socially acceptable ways, as an athlete, his aggressiveness has served him well. He has mastered every one of his extreme sports.

Lew has also written and published the story, "And Chocolate Shall Lead Us." This is a story about the consequences of global warming and climate change. The narrative includes recommendations to help us combat the consequences of this major problem. In this story there are four commandments to help save our planet.

The first: To find the truth, God, the one — look within yourself not to religions, myths, and legends.

The second: Select only leaders who can pass a rigorous test proving they have the people's best interest at heart.

The third: Do not burn fossil fuels: Use nuclear, wind, water and solar power.

The fourth: Knowledge, research and science will provide the answers. Have faith in rational thinking.

Although you may not agree with him, Lew presents clever and compelling points in this work, and he also has a children's version of the same story.

Dr. Hollander believes he has lived a charmed life. He cites two examples: It was 1984 and he was running the 100-mile Western States Run. He was hungry and between aid stations he reached into his shorts to pull out a sandwich. But it was soggy and dirty from sweat and it looked horrible. He decided to do the unscientific thing; he didn't think it through and discarded it. Then he criticized his decision. Unbelievably, within the next 100 yards, there, on the ground, he found a clean, wrapped sandwich dropped by someone ahead of him. So he thankfully satisfied his hunger.

Another example of Lew living a charmed life was during a recent Ironman in Hawaii. During the 112-mile bike ride, he realized he was violating one of the rules when he noticed a plug was missing from one of his handlebars. He didn't know how this could have happened, but he knew he was going to be disqualified if the officials noticed at the end of the ride that the handlebar was missing a plug. He began to stuff GU wrappers into his handlebar along with tape. Not satisfied with that, he remembered there was a local bike store a couple miles away. "I was having a nervous breakdown; I was so stressed not knowing what to do," remembers Lew. Then a short distance ahead he noticed a shiny handlebar plug on the ground. He stopped, picked it up, and it actually fit! "It was a miracle," Lew exclaimed, adding, ". . . and miracles continue to happen to me. Just like what Arnold Palmer said, 'The more I practice, the luckier I get.'"

Lew tells of another story that happened during one of his Hawaiian Ironman's. At about 10 miles into the run an attractive young woman 22-years-of-age gave him some water. She asked, "Do you want me to run with you?" As they ran together, she told him that her husband died about three months ago. Lew began thinking about his son Louis, who he thought would be a perfect fit for this woman, and he wanted to get her address. When they reached the finish line, Lew took her hand because he wanted to have their picture taken together. He didn't want to lose her. The next day when he looked at the photo, to his surprise he was the only one in the picture. He can't explain what happened. He calls the tale, "The Ghost Story."

I asked Lew what he wanted written on his tombstone. He said that he has been working on that for about 15 years and he's not sure just yet. He does know that he wants a proper resting place. He remarked that both of his parents were cremated and "they don't have a place." Lew said that his wife's family has a burial plot and he thinks that's a better idea.

In talking about his Ironman accomplishments, Lew said those goals were for personal ego gratification and that no one else cared. Being a scientist and making a contribution are far more important to him. That's Lew—Dr. Ironman. He has a realistic level of aspiration, plays like a kid, and uses his brain to research his activities.

XI

Life After the Western States Run

I began running on the trail again a few weeks after my 2002 Western States 100 triumph. I slowly increased the distance on my training runs, and then completed another Ride & Tie world championship. But I wasn't focusing on competing in the 2003 Western States Endurance Run; it definitely wasn't playing a major role in my mind.

Sometime in November I was talking to my sister Beverly on the phone and she brought up the subject of the 2003 Western States Run. I told her that I hadn't sent in an entry since I was totally undecided about running it again. One would think that by being undecided in November, it would be a major clue regarding my mental state about motivation and desire. Unfortunately, I didn't recognize my lack of strong motivation or properly assess my needs at the time. Beverly suggested that I enter the run anyway, so I could have the option of running or not running. Without giving it much thought, I entered. For me, that was a trap because if I enter something, then I'm going to do it. I can't simply pull out of an event without a substantial reason.

That year I decided to attend the Western States drawing unlike the previous year when I went to a party instead of to the lottery drawing. I parked my Chevy van in Cool that Saturday, and the plan was to run from Auburn to my house, and then back to my van, a total distance of approximately 28 miles. I spent maybe an hour or so at the drawing and then left to begin my run before the drawing was finished. This was another clue that I didn't recognize. Up to that point my name wasn't called. I then ran home, ate a sandwich, and headed back on the trail to pick up my van. As I was running back on the trail I met Diane Dixon-Johnson and Steve Rohm at about the 15-mile marker. Both Diane and

Steve were at the drawing and their entries were drawn in the lottery. As our paths crossed, Diane said to me, "You're in!"

My emotional response was disappointment. It's as though a cloud of dread had overcome me. Another major clue about my lack of motivation! And I paid for it later—a remarkable example of the defense mechanism of repression at work. I continued running to where I parked my van and felt as though I was running with my feet encased in cement. I certainly wasn't running like winged Mercury.

I trained for the run over the next few months and asked Chris Turney to assist me. We met one day a week at the Auburn High School track. Chris had me run a combination of laps at a fast pace and then do a series of stretching exercises. It obviously helped because I performed a personal best time of five hours and fifty-four minutes on the 50K Way To Cool Run, nine hours and six minutes for the 50-mile Jed Smith Run, and a ten hour and nine minute time on the 50-mile American River Run. These were by far my best times for these events. Chris talked about me running a 24-hour Western States time. My Ride & Tie friend, 40-something year old Jim Dempsey knocked over four hours off the finishing time on his second Western States Run. I clearly was not dealing with reality. I was having delusions of grandeur. However, I was running well.

In the middle of May I ran with my Ride & Tie friends Tom Christofk, Tony Brickel, Chris Turney, and others on a Wednesday night run. This run was traditional and long-standing. On this particular night the run was somewhere between seven to ten miles. We were about a mile-and-a-half to the finish and I was experiencing some difficulty with keeping my running shorts up. But that didn't stop me from racing Tom and Tony! I had never beaten them in any training run, but I felt pretty good and being the competitive person I am, I ran hard. I still didn't beat them, but I was very close. It was a moral victory for me.

The next day I paid for my moral victory; I could hardly walk. I made an appointment with chiropractor Matt Lambert, a runner, and talked to him about my condition. I damaged the major muscle in my quad and he suggested that I not run, but walk and ride a bike for rehabilitation, so I did. That weekend I had arranged to run a 50-miler at Quicksilver in San Jose. Bob Edwards and Steve Anderson were going to be my pacers but I had to scratch that plan.

On Memorial Day weekend there's always a Western States training run. I wasn't sure that I was going to be ready. It was either Thursday or Friday prior to Memorial Day weekend when I was on the trail walking and met Bill Johnson who was riding his horse 'Enterprise.' I told him that I wasn't sure about my ability to run and asked him if he would time me on a one-mile practice jog. My thought was that if I could cover the one mile in 18 minutes, I could participate in the 75 miles or so weekend training run. Don't ask me to explain my logic because I can't. I covered the mile within 18 minutes and went on to participate that weekend in the training run. The first two days of that 50-some-mile run went slowly. On the third day Jerome Beauchamp and I went out for a short five to six mile run.

I had about a one month window before the actual run and I did not use this month wisely. I was fearful that the injury had compromised my training and conditioning, therefore, I did not taper. I remember running with Jerome Beauchamp and telling him, "I'm not motivated about doing the run." I never dealt with my lack of underlying motivation, but how could I back out now? My sister was coming out from the East Coast to help crew for me, and I couldn't disappoint her! I felt stuck. Subconsciously I was scared, uncommitted, and ambivalent.

The race weekend arrived. To make matters worse, I spent the evening before the run shopping in Squaw Valley with my sister and my current girlfriend. This was the last thing I should've been doing Friday night. That year we had a hotel room with a loft and I wanted to go to bed early since I was tired from walking. Beverly wasn't tired so she watched television. I was concerned about the television noise and my rest (or lack thereof). I went to bed angry about a number of things, and didn't sleep well.

I was still upset and angry that Saturday morning. At about 25 to 30miles into the run near Robinson Flat I arrived at an aid station and immediately started yelling at my girlfriend. I certainly didn't need to be dealing with negative energy at that time but I was. My running time into Robinson Flat wasn't quite as fast as the previous year. I wasn't feeling great. I had a lot of negative thoughts, and wondered why I was doing this run.

About 16 miles or so later and just beyond Devil's Thumb I saw Mark Falcone and Les Nightingale sitting in chairs. They told me that they were done. I passed Steve Rohm and he was done. So now the thought of consciously stopping came to the forefront of my mind. Then I reached the Deadwood aid station and the volunteer there told me that I should stop consuming my electrolyte drink for a while since I was gaining weight (signifying kidney problems) and feeling lousy. I did not listen to her. I wasn't thinking very clearly at this point.

I had 55 or so miles to go. I finally reached Michigan Bluff and talked to my crew. They sensed my difficulty and arranged for a runner to pace me to the next aid station at Foresthill. During this seven-mile stretch I didn't realize that I wasn't able to stand up straight. Nor did I comprehend that I was using my hand and arm for balance to navigate the switchbacks because otherwise I would have probably fallen over. I'm still not sure how I had gotten so out of touch.

Eventually I reached Foresthill and met my two pacers, Jerome Beauchamp and Chuck Mather. I had to lean on them in order to stand up straight. I finally got it. I felt like crap, was unmotivated, and was willing to call it quits. We got to the aid station where my friend Kellie Holsey tried to comfort me. I drank some soup and said, "I've had enough." I pulled myself after 62 miles into the run.

We returned home and a couple of hours later I felt better. I didn't die. I was thoroughly disappointed about not completing the run though. Hindsight suggests that I didn't deal clearly and realistically with myself. The moral of the story is to pay attention to the clues. The clues were there, just waiting for me to listen to myself and recognize them.

Two other disappointments followed between the years 2003 and 2007. I entered Tevis two different years on my mare Gypsy. The first time she 'tied up' (azoturia) and was pulled at Red Star Ridge. The second time she was pulled for lameness at Last Chance, which was about 50 miles into the ride. Jim Steere's youngest daughter, Jennifer, was also pulled at Last Chance, and we shared the ride back to Foresthill with our horses safely tucked in the trailer. Gypsy's injury was minor, thank heavens, and three weeks later this tough mare received best condition at a Ride & Tie race in Oregon.

Between 2003 and 2007, I ran Way Too Cool and American River endurance runs. I also entered on Gypsy for the American River Ride, anticipating that it would help condition her for the Ride & Tie season. As it turned out, I had the distinction of completing the most American River endurance runs and endurance rides within the same year. My horseshoer Gordon Palmer informed me about my record-holding accomplishment, since he had held the record previously. Gordon had also completed the Tevis 11 times and had a Western States Run buckle as well. Even though we are roughly the same age, Gordon was unable to run anymore; I suspect that bending over while shoeing horses all those years had taken its toll.

During these years, Gypsy and I competed in a number of Ride & Tie events. Gypsy completed the most Ride & Tie miles by a horse in the years 2005 through 2008. To cap it off, Doyle Eggers and I came in first place in the Ride & Tie man/man division in the year 2006.

The world Ride & Tie championship race held in Fort Bragg was significant and memorable. Doyle and I were partners for that race and we rode one of Bob Edwards' horses for the event. This horse, however, had an irritation behind her elbow as a result of the girth rubbing her. We were at the start when I noticed how bad it was. Doyle and I decided to head back to Don Strong's trailer to get a sleeve to go over the girth strap to keep it from further irritating the rub. Don told us where the sleeve was located in his trailer and mentioned that we have to fit it to size. I found the sleeve; we made the necessary adjustment, and then proceeded back to the race start. Of course, by now we were in last place. Regardless of that setback, we managed to do extremely well. We passed numerous teams and finished in the middle of the pack. I was grateful that Doyle was a strong and competitive runner, that he was a good rider, and that the makeshift sleeve protected the horse.

Kurt Miller, a great runner, was my partner in the 75-mile Ride & Tie held at Swanton near Santa Cruz. Doyle was one of our crew members. Kurt and I ran a practice 30-mile Ride & Tie on Gypsy. Up to this point, Kurt had run about 20-some miles in his longest run. He was a good steady runner up to that distance. I told him that if he got into trouble I could run as far as necessary to help him out. I figured that Gypsy would do fine for that 75-mile distance since she had already completed a two-day hundred-mile endurance ride. I knew that it was going to be a push for Kurt, but he was a young 40 and he could handle it. As it turned out, we did have one minor difficulty. At about 30 miles or so there was a vet check where I dropped Gypsy off and continued running. It took a while for Kurt to catch me because he told me that Gypsy was a little off and they spent extra time at the vet check. I was concerned about her condition and luckily I found an endurance rider on the trail who could assess her gait, none other than Jim Steere, DVM. I asked Dr. Steere if he noticed any lameness. He said, "She looks fine to me." So on we rode. That story illustrates Jim Steere's character. Even though he was competing in the same event, he still had time to help me. Helping others and making sure the horse was all right exemplified who Jim was.

Kurt, Gypsy, and I did just fine for the rest of the ride. The last five to ten miles of the event were in heavy fog; that part of the trail is near the Pacific Ocean. The three of us stayed together until the finish. Our team did well.

On one of the American River endurance rides Gypsy and I did extremely well. Normally, I don't push her on endurance rides. On this particular ride, I often got off her back to run with her. I did it because it's good for me to run and I could "save her" for the long day. We were doing fine, and it was about 35 to 40 miles into the ride when I realized that we were in the top five. I don't think I was being too hard on her that day; everything just seemed to come together. And I'm proud to report that we came in fourth! A half-hour after crossing the finish line,

I presented her for best condition. I knew we did well, but I didn't wait for all the horses to be evaluated for best condition before I left for home. To my surprise and delight, the following week I was notified to pick up my best condition award at Echo Valley Farm and Ranch Supply. Not only did Gypsy receive the award for best condition horse, she also received the award for High Point. Simply put, Gypsy's vet scores on the ride were superior to the hundred or so other horses who raced that day.

Steve Anderson and I partnered for many Ride & Ties, and in 2007 we came in first place in the man/man division. Gypsy came in first for the most miles and points that year too. Jonathan Jordan and I partnered in 2008 and came in first place in the man/man division for the Ride & Tie Association, and once again Gypsy came in first for the most miles and points that year.

For the world Ride & Tie championship in San Diego, I entered with my neighbor Diana Lundy. Diana had run Western States a number of times and had good equestrian skills, but she liked to run more than ride. During this event, the weather was extremely hot and a number of teams had their horses pulled because of hydration or lameness issues. There were three loops and each of them ended up back at camp. For some reason, Diana made the wrong turn on the last loop. I was at the finish with Gypsy when I realized that Diana was nowhere in sight. So I headed back out and eventually found an exhausted Diana on the trail, where she admitted to making the logistical error. I helped her get on the horse, told her to head for the finish line, and I followed on foot. Even with all that extra drama (and miles for me and Gypsy), we came in seventh place overall.

At some point I decided to compete in the 100-mile Ride & Tie at Swanton. I figured that I had the right horse, Gypsy, and all I had to do was to find the right human partner for this brutal event. My partner had to be able to run about 50 miles and ride about 50 miles within a 24-hour period. After the 2007 Ride & Tie series, I got serious about this challenge. I thought more and more about it and became determined to enter. My plan was to get ready by running the Way Too Cool

50K, the Jed Smith 50K, and the American River 50-mile run. I would get Gypsy ready by entering her in the American River 50 endurance ride, the Quicksilver Ride & Tie, the world championship Ride & Tie, and a Ride & Tie in Oregon. The rest of the plan, obviously, was to find the right partner.

I chose Jonathan Jordan and he agreed to be my partner. His riding ability was unquestionably strong. In the previous year, he rode 500 or so miles in one cross-country horse event. Riding was his strong suit. He joined me on the Way Too Cool 50K run, which to that point had been his longest run.

I knew that the element of running was going to be our biggest challenge at the Swanton event. One has to know how to properly hydrate and eat during a 24-hour event. You have to know how to take care yourself. That's easy to say, but difficult to do in the heat of competition.

For the American River 50 mile endurance run, I asked Steve Anderson, Tracy Bakewell, and Tony Brickel to pace me. The plan was for Steve to run the last 25 miles or so, then to have Tracy join us for about 15 to 20 miles. Tony would pace me for the last four miles or so which included Cardiac Hill. Thankfully, the weather was not too extreme; it was neither especially cold nor especially hot during that long day. The first 20 miles traversed along the bike path starting at Sacramento State University. The bike path led to the fish hatchery at Lake Natoma. I ran fairly easily to that point. Then the trail running started and the race became more difficult. Steve was a very good pacer. We had a chance to talk and he was very responsive to my needs. He carried my jacket, filled my water bottles, and got food for me. My current girlfriend since the end of 2004, Linda Shaw, was at every aid station and gave me tremendous support.

Eventually, Tracy joined us. Her husband Scott and their two kids were also there. My running pace began to slow, but Tracy told me that I was doing well. Sometimes words help, but sometimes they don't. I appreciated the fact that both she and Steve were assisting me during this run, but at that point I was just getting tired, which was par for the course. I was happy that I could still put one foot in front of the other and continue to keep going, and make each cut-off time in the process.

The three of us reached the end of the running trail where we found Tony. Now all we needed to do was to climb until we reached the Cardiac Hill aid station. We were close to the finish but there was still more climbing to do. I knew the area, I knew this hill, and had done it before; I would certainly be happy when I was done. My name was announced over the loudspeaker as I crossed the finish line. I received my completion jacket and now I was really happy. I had finished this run!

We hung around at the finish line for a short while before saying goodbye. Linda, Steve and I returned to the house, had dinner, and cleaned up before Steve returned to Santa Clara. I always felt great after I completed these events, but there typically is another one on the horizon. I was scheduled for a Ride & Tie in San Diego the following week.

On Wednesday I got a call from my Denby High School football teammate Ed Budde. Ed asked if I was going to be near San Diego on the 18th of the month. I told him that as a matter-of-fact I was, and mentioned the Ride & Tie event. He invited me to an NFL reunion. Ed played for the Kansas City Chiefs for 13 years and was the president of the team's alumni association. His son Brad played for the Chiefs for nine years and he was going to be there too.

I flew to San Diego that Friday, picked up a rental car, and attended the NFL reunion with the Budde family. I danced with Carolyn, Ed's wife, met son Brad and all the former players that evening. From there I drove to Jonathan and Tara's Old McDonald Ranch in Alpine. In addition to their three boys, they had 14 horses, a couple of cows, roosters, pigs, goats, dogs, and of course, a boa in the house.

Jonathan and I left for the race on Saturday morning with his two horses, Chrissie and Flyer. Jonathan wasn't sure which horse we were going to use in the 25-mile Ride & Tie until after talking with the veterinarian who examined Chrissie and Flyer. We wound up using Chrissie. What I remember most about this Ride & Tie is that I felt tired during the event. I was happy to complete this race without getting hurt. I only had one more event to complete during the difficult month of April, thank goodness for that.

The only eventful episode during this race didn't happen to us, but happened to Melanie Weir and her horse. I remember hearing her horse galloping and whinnying frantically, and people yelling and screaming. I turned around and saw this charging Arabian galloping toward me, rider-less. I raised my arms to wave him off, but quickly determined that this horse wasn't about to slow down. I swiftly got out of the way so I wouldn't get trampled. Unfortunately for Melanie and her partner, they didn't complete the race but did get a large vet bill as a result of the horse's wounds.

The last event for April was the American River 50-mile endurance ride. There were some 25 miles of common trail for both the endurance ride and the ultra-run. The ride started in the Negro Bar area, crossed the American River, continued to Cool, and finished in Auburn. Nothing unusual happened during this long endurance ride. My horse Gypsy was doing fine even though the temperature was extremely hot. I was concerned about metabolic challenges and keeping my horse safe. I did not want her tying up (azoturia). This race was about her conditioning and her conditioning only. Remember, the big goal was the 100 mile Ride & Tie in August. We finished the race and Gypsy was terrific as usual. During this 50-mile endurance ride I often got off her back and led her while I ran in front of the mare. I protected my horse as much as I could. I was accomplishing all the necessary things in order to be successful in the big event in August.

On May 17, Gypsy and I teamed up with David De LaRosa, who was a vet assistant at a horse facility near Santa Barbara. He can run marathons in about three hours. At the Boston Marathon, his time was a little over three hours. The Friday before the race, the temperature at the campsite was extremely hot. Early Saturday, the temperature seemed near 100 degrees. This was the Quicksilver Ride & Tie. Steve Anderson was the race director and he changed the length of the course from 22 to 30 miles. There was some heated discussion prior to the start of the race; people were critical of (and mad about) the change in mileage. The trail had been marked, so no changes were made. For some reason we didn't start early, but rather later than usual.

It was getting hotter and hotter, and yet we didn't begin until after 9:00 a.m. David started off riding while I was on the ground, running up this long steep hill. I quickly found Gypsy tied to a tree branch. I got on her and started riding to catch up with David.

It took me a while to catch him because he runs fast. We then switched off back and forth. He rode and then ran. The exchanges between us worked well. The first aid station was about seven and a half miles into the race. As we were getting nearer to the aid station, we were in front of the pack and tied with the team of Tom Johnson, Rufus Schneider, and the horse Saamson. Tom had won the Western States 100 Mile Run three times, and Saamson had won the Tevis Cup and the best condition award at the Tevis, as well as the Haggin Cup. Rufus was a young, forty-something, fast, female runner.

Gypsy and I were getting tired and we had another seven and a half miles to go to reach the aid station and vet check. I had difficulty catching David because I was concerned about Gypsy. I eventually caught David and he rode Gypsy to the vet check.

I ran into the vet check and discovered that Gypsy's pulse and respiration were high, but she eventually met the criteria established by the veterinarian team. The veterinarian who examined Gypsy told me to take it easy with the mare because the conditions for this race were not good for the horses.

The next loop was a repeat of the last one. I took it easy with Gypsy; I acknowledged what the veterinarian said and took it to heart. I certainly didn't want my horse to be hooked onto an IV drip of ringers lactate. I didn't catch David for the next 15 miles because I wasn't going to push Gypsy at all. I didn't want her to wind up colicking. Because of this concern, I was often on the ground running alongside her, especially on the hilly and difficult sections of the trail. I kept thinking about my main goal this year, which was yet to come. I just wanted to finish this race.

We eventually reached the finish line where David was waiting for us. That day there were four horses with physical problems and many of them were hooked up to IVs before they were allowed to leave.

Jonathan and I teamed up for the World Ride & Tie championship that June. As it turned out, the veterinarian who evaluated Gypsy at the pre-ride examination reported that she had a sore back. He suggested that we switch to a different saddle pad, and warned us that at each vet check the rider was going to have to remove the saddle so he could check the mare's back to make sure she could continue.

Before the race, it was clear that we couldn't compete at top level because of the sore back issue. I considered getting a different saddle and saddle pad. We decided to use two saddle pads to protect Gypsy's back. I talked with Jonathan, discussed the options, and concluded that this was a training event only. In other words, we were not going to push her, and this was ground time for us both.

That cautionary approach turned out to be good for Gypsy and Jonathan. As a result of the veterinary observation, Jonathan, Gypsy, and I did an eight and a half hour slow race. It was great conditioning for the two of them. Perfect! Incidentally, her back was fine at the conclusion of the ride. One more Ride & Tie event loomed in July before the 100-mile event in August.

I talked with Sue Smyth about doing a 30-mile Ride & Tie called Bandit Springs in Oregon. Sue had done Ride & Tie previously and was just getting back into the sport. She was not confident about her ability to run the distance required, and commented, "I didn't train enough." I told her if need be I would do most of the running, that was my mindset. We did some practice Ride & Ties before we headed to Oregon. At that Ride & Tie event, there was one big loop. We were second going into the vet check at about 15 miles into the race. At that point in the race we were doing just fine. Shortly after the vet check, I saw the first place horse tied to a tree with no runners in sight. I instantly knew that team had a problem, they ran by their horse. So now Sue, Gypsy, and I were in first place.

About three miles from the finish I tied Gypsy and ran ahead. After a while, I expected to see Sue and Gypsy, but they were nowhere in sight. There was an endurance ride taking place on the same trail, and I asked various riders who passed me if they had seen a woman in blue tights. Everybody said, "No."

I ran to the finish line, ate and drank. I then headed back on the trail, looking for my horse and Sue. Eventually I found them. Sue claimed, "I made a wrong turn and went an extra five miles or so." We finally finished. Our team did great and Gypsy got to complete more miles. It was onto the Swanton Pacific to compete in the 100-mile Ride & Tie.

My training and conditioning were basically completed. I was feeling super, didn't have any injuries, and was prepared. Gypsy had completed all the events appropriate for her conditioning. All I had to do was keep her sound and rested. For us, our training was done. I talked with Jonathan frequently about his conditioning. I repeatedly told him to run slow, long distances. At this point in time there was no need for speed training. Endurance and stamina were our significant keys to success

XII

The Third Hurdle: The 100-Mile Ride & Tie

The Swanton Pacific began as an endurance ride known as the Castle Rock Ride. The head veterinarian for that 50-mile ride suggested that the west region of the American Endurance Ride Conference (AERC) needed additional 100-mile endurance rides. That veterinarian was none other than Jim Steere. As the result of Dr. Steere's input, Ellen's parents, Lud and Barbara McCrary, set out in the spring of 1983 to create a 100-mile endurance ride in the northern Santa Cruz and southern San Mateo counties. To create the trail they explored the Pescadero Creek watershed, the village of Loma Mar, the Rancho Del Oso and the Butano and Big Basin state parks.

It was extremely helpful that the McCrary family were owners of Big Creek Lumber, a logging company that logged in the Butano Creek watershed and the surrounding areas. They knew that area as well as the backs of their hands. Lud and Barbara would go out on a weekend to picnic and explore old abandoned logging roads once used by their company. They finally located a potential trail route, and then the challenge really began. First, they had to restore flood-damaged roads and bridges that had been left idle for 45 years.

They came upon an opening in the forest that was covered in black caused by the tannic acid from the redwood bark. Their conversation went back and forth something like this: "Do we need a saw? Do we need a bulldozer? No. We need a boat." They referred to that particular area as "The Black Lagoon."

This Black Lagoon was not used as a through route for many years until their logging crews built a road around it. Bridges and routes need repairs each year. Originally logs were stacked at 90 degree angles in order to accomplish bridge repair. Each log layer was topped off with about six feet of soil. After 45 years these bridges were disintegrating and falling apart. They had to find a way around the bridges until their logging crew could build a new, strong bridge. A solution came to mind: Use a railroad flat car as a bridge. That brilliant idea worked. Another bridge was full of holes and it had to be patched every year. One bridge became The Wheel Barrow Bridge because a wheel barrel was used to transport gravel, rocks, and sand for repairs. They also installed a water trough named Sweet Water Gulch. They eventually upgraded the original trail into a drivable logging road and then it became easier for them to maintain that road.

There was a lot of know-how and hard labor to be done in order to create this endurance ride. Luckily, they had the money, time, energy, will, creativity, ingenuity, intelligence, persistence, and labor to successfully complete the job. As a result, the Swanton Pacific 100 came to be in 1983.

The Swanton Pacific 100 hosted the first-ever international 100 mile endurance ride in the Western Hemisphere sanctioned by the Federation Equestre Internationale. Riders from Europe, Canada, Australia, and New Zealand entered. The Swanton Pacific created history. As the years passed they initiated a 75-mile endurance ride using roughly the same trail system. In 2008 it was the Swanton Pacific's Silver Anniversary. Unfortunately, it was also its last ride because Barbara and Lud retired. Daughter Ellen now tells us about the origins of the one-and-only 100 mile Ride & Tie.

In 1983, Kathy DeVito and Melinda Creel tested the idea of doing a 100-mile Ride & Tie. These two gutsy and tough women of this woman/woman team entered along with endurance riders and completed the Swanton Pacific in 22 hours and 37 minutes on their horse Sur Nefix.

The following year, Warren Hellman found a partner crazy enough to attempt that ride and his name was Pat Browning. Pat's motivation was plain and simple. His goal was to beat the girl's completion time. Pat and Warren were successful; their finishing time was 20 hours and eight minutes. Pat recalled that he was extremely happy with their success. The 100-mile Ride & Tie requires a unique combination of runner, rider and horse.

It wasn't until 1996 that Dennis Rinde (who finished 7th place twice at the Boston Marathon and just missed making the Olympic trials) revived the idea and stirred up interest. In 1996, the Swanton Pacific became the first officially sanctioned 100-mile Ride & Tie. Jim Steere, head veterinarian for the Swanton Pacific 100-mile endurance ride, supported the concept of the 100-mile Ride & Tie. He came up with the vet criteria for the horse. Ellen Rinde, race manager, established human race criteria and limited the entries to 10 teams. One criterion for the humans was at least one team member must have successfully completed a 100-mile endurance ride or a five-day 250-mile endurance ride. Jonathan Jordan, Gypsy, and I all met race criteria. We entered that ride in 2008.

On August 15, 2008 Linda Smith (a friend), Linda Shaw (my fiancée at the time), Gypsy, and I arrived at the race site, a small community of Davenport near Santa Cruz, California. We parked the rig and started to look for Jonathan. We eventually found him driving on one of the nearby roads but going in the wrong direction. Unfortunately, this would foreshadow what was to come. We redirected Jonathan and then headed back to the horse camp.

In addition to our 100-mile Ride & Tie event there were the 75-mile Ride & Tie and a 100-mile and 75-mile endurance rides taking place at the same time. We took Gypsy to the initial vet check and she passed with flying colors. So we were ready to go. Race director Ellen Rinde scheduled a race meeting for only the Ride & Tie teams that evening. There were a total of three teams entered in the 100-mile Ride & Tie. This meant there were four "crazy" people besides Jonathan and me. There's no doubt that this race scares people because of its difficulty. The other two teams had participants from Utah. One man, Dr. Bruce Burnham, had completed this event before with Jim Dempsey. His partner that year was a female whom I didn't know. Bruce had completed 100-mile endurance runs as well as 100-mile endurance rides and was no stranger to Ride & Tie. As a matter of fact, Bob Edwards, a mutual friend and I were his pacer a few years earlier on the American River 50-mile endurance run.

The other team consisted of a young veterinarian and her "Tevis man" friend. He wore a Tevis buckle to hold up his jeans. At the meeting we agreed to meet on the trail for an early starting time Saturday morning. That evening we ate an early dinner and made sure Gypsy had plenty to eat; the next day was going to be long. A more accurate statement would be a long day and a long night. I realized that we were not going to beat Tom Christofk's and Dan Barger's record time of 17-plus hours. My goal was simply to complete the ride. I wasn't too concerned about how long it would take. I did know that it was going to be a long 24 hours (completion criteria) and I prayed that Jonathan was rested and ready. I knew that Gypsy and I were ready. Hopefully we'd get through the day and night in one piece.

The three Ride & Tie teams were scheduled to meet on the trail prior to the starting time of the race. Jonathan and I arrived around 4:30 a.m., the agreed upon and official starting time. The other two teams were nowhere to be found. We began walking up the trail to allow the other two teams to catch us. When they caught us, the race would begin. They did catch us, and the adventure started! This was typical of the sportsmanship of Ride & Tie competitors.

Glow Sticks marked the trail with light emanating from these tubes so the trail was clear to the rider and runner. Remember, horses have night vision. At that time in the morning it was cool, and we all felt great. Of course, the one thing that was common during a long race was the change in a competitor's feeling. In other words, you didn't feel great all the time nor did you feel lousy all the time. So, if you were not feeling great you knew it would likely change, and thank goodness for that; no one wants to feel lousy all the time.

We were in the lead until one of the younger teams from Utah passed us. This team was the Tevis buckle guy with the veterinarian female partner. It was early in the race and being in second place was okay at that point. The Swanton Pacific was primarily an endurance ride which meant that some of the faster riders passed us and made comments such as, "Good luck", "You look great," "Way to go," and "Where's the horse?" Melissa Ribley, the endurance and Ride & Tie veterinarian, Cathy Scott, Matt Maderios, and Warren Hellman were some of those riders.

After the first aid station, we were still in second place. Then we proceeded on a single-track trail with Jonathan running ahead. When I caught him, he was helping the veterinarian with her horse. He called out, "Continue riding and tie farther down the trail." Now we were in the lead and things were still going great. My worry was directed toward making the upcoming vet check cut-off time. This vet check was about 35 miles into the Ride & Tie. Making cutoffs in the running of Western States, Tevis, and in this race was extremely important. If you didn't make it, you were pulled out of the race.

We arrived at the 35-mile vet check in first place; I was pleased. Gypsy passed the veterinary evaluation and we allowed her to eat and rest. She was good at protecting herself, and relaxed and closed her eyes during rest periods. We wolfed down pancakes brought by the two Linda's. Jonathan and I each had a Linda as personal crew. The other two Ride & Tie teams eventually arrived at the vet check and appeared to be all there together. We left the vet check before our competitors, so we were still in first place.

The next vet check was located at the Butano airstrip at the 50-mile marker. During the next 15-mile stretch we managed to keep up with several endurance riders, some of whom I knew. It was terrific to be running and riding while keeping up with somebody who was only riding. I frequently asked Jonathan, "Are you eating, are you drinking?" and cautioned him to take care of himself. By this time, the hills seemed tougher and longer, and I began to wonder how much longer before we arrived at the next vet check. The temperature in the mountains during this time of day was hot. Hot is probably in the mid to upper 90s.

The vet check was now in sight and our strategy had been for me to bring Gypsy into the vet check and get her through the evaluation. I knew my horse better than anyone, so that was the plan we used. It was important for both Jonathan and Gypsy to eat and drink. I was taking care of my 68-year-youthful body and I kept reminding my 50-year-old-plus partner, to do the same. It was important for us to physically recover and refuel so that we had the energy to go on. I couldn't stress this enough and probably sounded like a broken record, but this was one of the keys to a successful completion of a strenuous, all-day event.

The next aid station was Lud's at approximately 55 miles, where he had water for the horses and goodies for the participants. Standing near Lud, I heard him talking on the radio with the people at the prior vet check. He told us that the other two teams from Ride & Tie had been pulled. They did not make the cutoff time. I wondered if something could be wrong with the horses or with them, or all six.

Now, not only were we in the lead, but our competition had bit the dust. I must admit that was okay because now I didn't have to worry about the other two teams.

It was very important for us to protect Gypsy as well as ourselves in order to get through this event. To motivate Jonathan in a positive way, I'd make statements like, "You only have to ride about 22 miles and run another 22 miles for us to finish." I never asked him if those comments made a difference. Of course we'd already been running and riding for about 10 to 12 hours. I had no qualms about Jonathan's ability to ride the remaining distance. The previous year he rode a Pony Express ride that covered over 50 miles a day for eight continuous days. He was a terrific rider, extremely knowledgeable horseman, and had a tough and seasoned butt. However, I was concerned about his ability to run the distance because it was uncharted territory for him. Up to that point, a 50K had been his longest run. This would be his longest run and his first 24-hour event.

In a Ride & Tie event like this, a human has to be able to hydrate, electrolyte, urinate, eat properly, and get rid of human waste during the 24-hour race. The humans also have to take care of the horse and monitor it to make sure the animal eats, drinks, urinates, ingests the necessary electrolytes, and has bowel movements. It's critical for the horse to pass each vet check without lameness or metabolic issues. If the horse can't continue, the whole team is pulled. Often during an event like this, the human body begins to shut down, which can also happen to the horse. And when our body begins to shut down, we don't think about food and are not interested in eating or drinking. Nothing tastes good at that point. You can't get through these events without the necessary calories for fuel. It's like a car. The car has to have fuel in the tank. The runner has to have fuel in his or her tank too.

The next vet check was at about 70 miles. The Linda's were there waiting for us. They were terrific and did a tremendous and competent job. They had freshly cooked hamburgers and drinks available, and made sure the horse had a mash of beet pulp and supplements to eat, in addition to hay and water. Both Linda's were concerned about Jonathan and commented that he sounded strange and didn't appear too interested in eating. So for the last two vet checks, they attempted to get him eating.

Just prior to the Sawmill vet check, I was riding Gypsy on a very steep switchback trail. In fact, it was so steep that my saddle slipped forward and I started to slide up on Gypsy's neck. I grabbed her neck with both arms so I wouldn't fall off and plummet down the steep drop off. I wasn't limber enough to swing either my right or left foot over the saddle to get off the mare. I yelled at Jonathan and with a huge amount of panic and anxiety in my voice told him to come back and help me get off Gypsy. He ran back to help, and I'm glad to report that the situation had a happy ending. One might think I would be embarrassed, but no, I was just pooped. Once on the ground, I adjusted the saddle properly. Thank goodness no one was injured and Jonathan was near enough to hear my call of distress.

We were in the dark of night but still doing well. This meant we were going in a forward direction. I was certainly tired, but still motivated. When I was on the ground and not in the saddle, I simply put one foot in front of the other, over and over and over. You rested when you were in the saddle. You could really rest when the race was over.

At about 85 miles, we passed Steve Anderson who was helping out by manning a mini aid station. He was also in charge of opening and closing the gate because of all the grazing cattle in the area. It was pitch dark and the thick ocean fog had rolled in. Jonathan and I were near each other; I was running while Jonathan was riding. At one point Jonathan said he needed to go to the bathroom, so I took Gypsy and told him that I would continue walking and he could catch up with us.

I looked back for Jonathan every few minutes, expecting to see the light from his LED. No such luck. I began to worry. Now here was my dilemma: One unwritten rule in Ride & Tie is that you must always keep going forward to reach the next vet check and then wait for your partner there. However, I thought that Jonathan might be injured. He might have cramped up, fallen down, and been unable to get to his feet. What if he couldn't move? What if he was really sick? Thoughts like these raced through my mind.

I didn't go back. The unwritten rule of Ride & Tie took precedence and I continued down the trail. Remember, it was pitch-dark and I was following Glow Sticks. Gypsy and I went through a wooded area, crossed a stream, leapt across railroad tracks, and trotted by ranches. I was still walking and leading my horse down the trail when a couple of endurance riders passed me. I asked, "Have you seen my partner Jonathan? He's on foot." They all said, "No."

After about a half an hour the drag riders eventually caught me. Drag riders follow all the endurance riders at the back of the pack, making sure no one is lost or in trouble. Should there be an issue, they are there to help. Of course there were no drag riders for us Ride & Tie competitors. I also asked them if they had seen Jonathan, with the same "no" as a reply. Aside from worrying about Jonathan and his possible condition, I am ashamed to say that my thoughts also pertained to completing this ride. Gypsy and I had gone approximately 90 miles and were about 22 hours into the race. We might not have finished. Of course this was minor compared to anything horrible that could have happened to Jonathan.

Finally, Gypsy and I arrived at the vet check. We were at about the 93-mile marker. I told both Linda's that I hadn't seen Jonathan for a long time. All three of us were now worried. I told the veterinarian that I thought my partner was lost or hurt, and described where I last saw Jonathan. The vet was from the area, knowledgeable, and told me that the drag riders had just pulled all the Glow Sticks. So if Jonathan was still on the trail, he was without benefit of Glow Sticks to follow. How could he ever find his way in the dark with the maze of intersections of all those trails?

The vet and a couple of volunteers drove out and replaced at least some Glow Sticks. A few minutes later, after the vet and volunteers had left, Jonathan arrived! I still don't understand how he accomplished this feat. And what I didn't mention to anyone were the thoughts of how I would break the news to Tara about Jonathan's demise.

The vet came back and called out for us to get on that horse and complete the ride. "What are you two waiting for?" he hollered. Jonathan remarked that he was scared to death and he ran with his head pointed downward, looking for trail signs to assist him. I was still not sure of everything that happened to him that evening, but we proceeded and Jonathan was lollygagging with the attractive female drag riders from the endurance ride. I can only guess what he was talking about. I yelled at Jonathan, "Let's get going so we can finish this ride!"

We completed the 100-mile Ride & Tie the morning of August 17, 2008. I took Gypsy through the vet check, she passed, and I tucked her into a small portable corral where she could rest and eat. Linda and I spent some intense time talking about the event. I was exhausted, sore, and yet hyper. I got some rest before the morning awards presentation. We attended the awards breakfast where we mingled with all the competitors and of course shared stories about our triumphant ordeal. In the late morning we packed up and headed for home after saying all our goodbyes.

Now I had completed three major, unique, and physically difficult events, the 100-mile Western States Run, the 100-mile Ride & Tie, and the 100-mile Tevis Cup. I'm one of only four individuals in the world to have completed these three events. Further, I am the oldest person to have completed these events while in his 60s. I was proud and extremely grateful that I had wonderful partners in Jonathan and Gypsy, and a great crew. But Gypsy and I were not finished yet as the year wasn't over; it was only August.

The next Ride & Tie was September 13th and was called The Coolest Run, Ride & Tie. Linda and I were the race directors for the event in our hometown of Cool. Jim Steere was our head veterinarian. We had our usual elaborate potluck on Friday evening, the race on Saturday, and the awards luncheon that followed. My race partners were Josh Steffen, a 20-something-year-old who had enlisted in the Air Force, and of course Gypsy. Josh wanted to get flight training from the Air Force, and become a commercial airline pilot after leaving the service. I met Josh a couple years before at our Ride & Tie event. I remember seeing him run on the trail and thinking to myself, "Wow, he's fast!" One of my crew members and dear friend, Gary Ireland, introduced me to Josh at that event since our horse trailers were parked adjacent to each other.

I had called Josh a couple of times after that meeting; I was looking for a race partner. Our schedules didn't mesh until 2008 when Josh told me he would be delighted to be my partner. We set up a practice Ride & Tie, and much to my surprise I watched as he simply vaulted onto Gypsy's back, no need for putting a foot in the stirrup. He ran like the wind. We talked about training and his college running experience. We also talked about VO2 formulas, recovery and pacing. After our practice, I knew we were very likely to win the 22-mile event. He was exceptionally fast, an extremely good rider, and also owned a horse named Gypsy. He remarked that his mom Kim was an endurance rider, a massage therapy practitioner, and that she would come to the event and help crew. We made plans to meet the morning of the race.

Josh started out on Gypsy (my Gypsy) while I was on the ground running. We did an exchange and were doing fine for the first three miles or so until my left stirrup fell to the ground. I needed to make a lightning fast decision: Do I stop my horse and retrieve the stirrup or do I continue riding minus a stirrup? I made the decision to continue riding. I had no idea if it was the right decision at the time.

It was a little over four miles into the ride when Gypsy and I reached a creek crossing. That's where two women from the Androtti family team passed us. Remember, I could only use one stirrup and that limited how fast we could travel. When we galloped the hills, almost my entire weight was on the right side of the horse, with my right leg braced in the remaining stirrup. Obviously my balance wasn't terrific and I didn't want to be hard on Gypsy's back and possibly hurt her. We were definitely at a disadvantage. One of the Androtti girls galloped hard and fast up that steep hill, leaving us in the dust. These girls were fast and were now in the lead. Within a half a mile or so, Gypsy and I reached the 5-mile aid station.

As I approached the station, I started screaming, "I lost my stirrup—does anybody have a stirrup?" Greg Kimler, my Tevis buddy and one of our great sponsors, and Barbara Mancia, were assisting at the aid station. Barbara quickly responded, "I have a saddle in my horse trailer; I'll take off the stirrup and let you use it." We took precious minutes to make the necessary adjustment. In this race every minute counts. I got back on Gypsy and we were back in the race, still in second place. I was now able to really compete since I got my balance back.

I arrived at the next aid station and told the story to the two Linda's, and to Kim, Josh's mother. We had just completed the first loop of nine miles and now faced a second loop of four miles. When I passed the Kimler and Mancia aid station the second time, they motioned me to stop. Melissa Ribley had retrieved my stirrup on the trail. I dismounted and tied the stirrup to my saddle. I decided to swap the stirrups at the next vet check.

The Linda's and Kim took care of Gypsy while I changed the stirrups. Tony Brickel also helped take care of Gypsy. Her pulse was too high to meet criteria, and therefore she couldn't successfully pass the vet check. The horse had to meet criteria before the rider could take the horse to the veterinarian for evaluation. It took Gypsy some time to recover before I could vet her through; meanwhile Josh was running ahead down the trail for the third and last loop. I became concerned because it was taking so long for Gypsy to recover while Josh was out on the trail running. The temperature was in the 90s and Gypsy was tired; so was Josh. I was somewhat rested since I was mostly riding. Finally, Gypsy met the pulse and respiration criteria and she was vetted through.

I believed that we were in second place at that moment. I finally reached Josh and found him exhausted and whipped, to say the least. Just because he was a 20-something-year-old kid didn't mean he could run all day in the hills and in the heat. We made the necessary exchanges and continued without any more incidents. Josh was out of gas, but still moving in the right direction. We reached the finish line in less than three hours for 22 miles, placing second. We passed the vet examination and then found out that the Andretti girls had a major problem. Jim Steere pulled their horse due to lameness. We won!

Gypsy had come through again. We won the man/man division, Melissa Ribley and Cathy Scott won the woman/woman division, and Jonathan Jordan and Carrie Barrett won the man/woman division. Jonathon's horse Flyer won the coveted best conditioned award. The year so far was going great.

There was a Ride & Tie scheduled on September 21st called the Californios Tejon Fandango. If I had been thinking clearly, I would've decided to give my horse a rest, but I wasn't thinking properly, and teamed up with Steve Anderson for this ride. The base camp was located at the historic Tejon Ranch, the oldest private ranch in California.

The race started on Sunday morning. I was riding Gypsy while Steve was running. About five miles out I started losing the damned stirrup. Not again! Luckily there was a ranch hand on the trail and we used string and duct tape to make the necessary repair. So far on this ride, there were plenty of steep, and then downhill trails. Steve and I made ties and were doing okay even though we lost some time with the stirrup issue. Maybe after eight to ten miles, I noticed that Gypsy was off on her left front and looked pretty lame. This was not good.

Steve ran ahead while I walked with Gypsy toward the vet check, some two to five miles down the trail. When we reached the vet check, Gypsy was truly lame. We were out of the race. Gypsy got a trailer ride back to base camp, where I got another vet evaluation, gave her Butte (an analgesic and anti-inflammatory drug), and wrapped her leg. I was thoroughly disappointed and discouraged. I knew I had made a major mistake by going to this ride. Gypsy needed time off, and I didn't give it to her. We got back home and the next morning I called Kris Bartow, my vet.

Kris performed a thorough examination and suggested I take Gypsy to the vet clinic at University of California at Davis so they could take X-rays and ultrasound scans of her leg to determine the degree of damage. The diagnosis was that she had minor ligament damage and mild tendonitis. The treatment was to wrap her leg for a few weeks and then hand-walk her, starting with five minutes at a time. Her rehab began, and there would be no competitions for Gypsy for the rest of the year. This was the end of September.

My 50th reunion at Denby High School in Detroit, Michigan, was in October and I wanted to see my old friends. I began thinking about when I was a senior in 1957, when I played offensive guard and defensive middle guard on the football team. In those days, Denby was a football powerhouse. This reunion was held on Saturday in the town of Sterling Heights near Detroit. I planned on meeting my high school teammate Ed Budde and his wife Carolyn and other friends from the football team. I flew into Detroit on Friday.

That first night I spent with my cousin Steve Lasser reminiscing about old times. I showed him a picture of me and Ed, taken by one of the major Detroit newspapers, the Detroit Free Press. I had made a copy of that picture so I could give it to Ed. That picture was taken when we were selected as co-linemen of the week. Each week the Detroit Free Press selected a story from one of the high school football games. In that particular game against Central, I blocked a punt, made a couple of quarterback sacks, and recovered a fumble. When the picture was taken at the newspaper offices, Ed wore his practice jersey and I wore a game day jersey. That picture never appeared in the paper, but I had a copy. I was going to surprise Ed with the picture. I went out for a run that morning and then Steve and I had brunch at a deli near his home. Then I headed for Sterling Heights to attend the reunion.

I checked into the motel and recognized some classmates in the lounge area. I went to my room, got cleaned up, turned on the radio and listened to the Saturday game between the University of Michigan and Toledo. I was shocked that Michigan lost to Toledo that day. That might have been the greatest football upset in college history! After the game I called Ed's room and we planned to meet downstairs.

Ed, Carolyn and I met and then I presented him with the picture before going to the reunion. Ed was surprised and pleased by my gift, and apparently didn't remember the photo until I reminded him of the story.

I found my good friend Dr. Wayne Fisk at the reunion. Wayne and I had been friends for such a long time, and I was happy that we kept in contact. In fact, we were both psychologists and attended the same graduate school together at Wayne State University. I hadn't seen Wayne since my mother's death and the unveiling of her headstone in 2002.

Ed and Carolyn, Bob Budde and his wife, Larry Hudas and his wife, Ron Transik, Mitchell Newman and I were seated at the players' table. There were so many memories of the 1957 football season and most of them were terrific.

The day after the reunion, I visited my buddy Wayne Fiske before going to the airport. We discussed the reunion and the conflicting emotions it prompted. I talked about the likelihood of not seeing my former high school classmates ever again. It was difficult to believe that we were at this age. For the most part, many friends and acquaintances still looked good. I would like the reunions to go on forever, just seeing and being with those people brought back many fond memories. In fact, most of the memories are great. Ernest Becker wrote a book titled "The Denial of Death" and it fits me.

Looking back at my high school years, I remember various conflicts. I do not do well with authority figures, I don't like rules and regulations, and I remembered my high school counselor telling me in front of my parents that I had to grow up. I distinctly remember that sentence, and it's been with me for over 50 years. I know what he meant. Take responsibility for your actions, do your best, be decent to others and to yourself. Maybe in some ways I have grown up. In some ways I have not. Back then I was perceived as being a greaser, smart, and tough. Today, the perception might be that I am smart and tough. I don't think I'm perceived as a greaser. I often think of myself as being 17 and an eternal teenager. It can be difficult to think of one's self as getting old.

XIII

2009: A Turning Point

The year 2009 was another turning point in my life, to put it mildly. I'll start with Gypsy. She had been rehabilitated during the last three months of 2008 as a result of her tendonitis injury. She had a clean bill of health and I was ready to bring her conditioning back to where it was before her injury. It was now January 2009 and I began thinking about the Ride & Tie events for the upcoming year. I called my veterinarian Kris Bartow, a young fifty-something, and asked him about teaming up for the world championship in June. He said he needed to run more to get in shape for the event. We talked about his running and us getting together for some practice Ride & Ties. With all these thoughts looming about competition, it was time to get on Gypsy's back and ride her again.

On a cold but dry Thursday morning in late January, just prior to Super Bowl Sunday, Linda and I decided to take the two horses out on a conditioning ride near our home in Cool, located on the Wendell Robie Trail (named after the founder of the Western States Trail Foundation, the organization that hosts the Tevis each year). It was time to start conditioning Gypsy at a trot in order to get her ready and in racing shape. I was mounted on Gypsy and Linda was riding Raider. Both horses were excited, snorting, and anxious to go. Gypsy and I were in the lead, and Linda and Raider were close behind. We had just passed the 17-mile marker on the trail when Linda shouted at me to slow down because Raider was being difficult.

A mere moment after Linda yelled, Gypsy bucked, and it was quite a wild-horse-rodeo buck. I was launched out of the saddle, flew through the air, and landed on my back with a resounding thud. I knew instantly I was in trouble. I was afraid to move a muscle, and wasn't quite certain that I could even if I wanted to. This was serious, and I knew it. Linda wanted to move me off the trail and I told her in no uncertain terms, "Don't touch me. Don't move me." Fortunately, she had a cell phone with her and dialed 911. Eventually, she was able to make contact and I told her that our location was between the 17 and 17-1/2 mile marker. I didn't lose consciousness, but I was in significant pain. Linda attempted to put gloves on my hands to keep me warm, but my hands and fingers were too sensitive and too swollen. She stripped her horse of his gear and placed the saddle blanket over me. She wanted to keep me warm, out of shock, and as comfortable as possible. Linda was great; she's a wonderful woman who knew just what to do.

A runner friend, Rick Valentine, happened to be out for a run and stumbled over us on the trail. Linda sent him to find help. After maybe half an hour, I heard the sound of a helicopter overhead. Everyone knows that distinct sound. A rescue crew on foot arrived about a half hour later. It seems they got lost and went in the wrong direction on the trail, which is easy to do if you don't know the terrain. Someone from the rescue crew placed a brace on me to support my head and neck; I was now stabilized.

The helicopter was unable to land because of the density of the forest, but luckily Gypsy bucked me off where there happened to be a tree opening. As a result, the helicopter was able to drop a line near the accident spot on the trail. After being placed on the sling, they zipped me up in a canvas body bag, only I was alive. They made sure that I closed my eyes to protect them from the wind the helicopter blades created and before I knew it, I was lifted in the air. It was such a strange sensation to be hauled up into the air like that, and I was so glad I wasn't swinging around wildly. I heard the roaring sound of the helicopter surrounding me.

After what seemed like a short distance, the helicopter landed somewhere. I didn't have any idea where I was, even though I knew the area well. I was then taken out of the body bag, placed inside the helicopter and flown towards the hospital.

Now on the ground, off we travelled again. I was asked a series of questions to evaluate my state of consciousness; I was fully conscious.

But of course, I wasn't moving at that point. We arrived at a destination which turned out to be the trauma center at the hospital. I was immediately transferred to a gurney and taken somewhere in the hospital. I talked briefly to a doctor and then found myself alone, staring at the ceiling. Even after talking to a couple of nurses, I still didn't know what was happening. I was wondering all kinds of things. I knew I could still wiggle my toes and I practiced that over and over determining I was not paralyzed. Well, at least I was praying that I wasn't paralyzed.

Someone came in and began carrying on a conversation with me. At first I thought it was a doctor, but soon realized that it was my friend Bill Johnson. I talked with him but don't remember what I said, or for that matter what he said. Finally, a medical technician wheeled me to another location. On the way to wherever we were going, another friend Kevin Doyle showed up and we talked briefly. Once again, I don't remember what was said. My gurney landed in a room where I was to have a series of scans, and the technician told me not to move. After all the scans and X-rays were taken, I was finally transported to my private room at the orthopedic center at Sutter Roseville Hospital where I was diagnosed with a broken neck.

It seemed like just a short few moments before I was joined by Linda, Michael Raposselli, and my daughter Lori. I was surprised that Michael was there but even more shocked to see Lori. She had been angry with me for some time and we had not spoken in quite a while. If you break your neck, it seems, things can change. Lucky me, I could now begin to work on a relationship with my daughter. You might ask what good can come of a broken neck. Well, in my case it worked to my advantage.

As it turned out, I had broken the processes bones that help stabilize the neck. But I also found out that I had stenosis, a narrowing of my spinal cord. I never would have known of this condition without my trip to the hospital that day. 'Family' certainly took on a whole new meaning. Some people believe that things happen for a reason, I believe that we can also create our own reasons, but random events do come into play.

The orthopedic surgeon finally showed up while I was talking on the phone to my brother Ron, a physician, who lived in Maryland. I quickly handed the phone to the surgeon so he could talk to my brother. After he finished I got back on the phone; Ron wasn't impressed with the doctor, but it's not uncommon for Ron to be unimpressed with another doctor. If you knew my brother, you would know what I mean. My treatment was simply morphine coupled with a head and neck brace, while lying on my back. I sucked on ice and was hooked up to an IV. The doctor did not have the entire test results at this juncture.

Friday came along and it was pretty much the same story. I was not in any pain but I still felt uncomfortable. I was grateful Linda was there. At one point I was given broth and then spit it out. It seemed that the morphine was upsetting my stomach and I couldn't hold food down. Linda left for the evening after witnessing my so-called eating experience. She said she would return on Saturday afternoon. That entire day was really a blur.

It was now early Saturday morning, and I was extremely uncomfortable. I simply could not get the nurses and aides to properly take care of me, causing me to be extremely agitated and irritable. I was becoming more and more aware of my limitations, which—as you can well imagine, really bothered me.

Later that morning, a physical therapist arrived at my bedside. The morphine treatment had ended so I finally got to eat breakfast. The physical therapist said she was going to get me out of bed so I could walk. I remember being terrified to move and panicked at the idea of walking. I remember saying to her repeatedly, "Are you sure that I should get out of bed?" Before I knew it I had my feet on the floor. I was wearing my neck harness, which I later found out was to be my friend 24/7. She directed me with, "Stand, hold onto my hand, and I'll help you begin to walk."

The nurse's station was a triangle-like configuration. Surrounding the perimeter of the station were patient rooms, with a nice wide walkway between the rooms and the station. So now I had an indoor track to maneuver and navigate in and around. The distance around this track was between 300 and 400 feet. It didn't take me long, thank goodness, to realize that my walking wasn't impaired. I just had to be upright when I turned my head, and do it in unison with my body and shoulders. I was limber so this wasn't going to be a problem. I took several laps with the physical therapist and she finally commented, "You're doing fine. I have to go, so why not get the nurses to walk with you." I replied, "Fine." So now I had another pacer, a friendly nurse. After just a few short minutes, this nurse said, "I'll just sit down and watch you do your laps." I walked and I walked, and I walked some more because I didn't want to go back to bed.

A trauma surgeon entered my 'indoor track' area and was reviewing patient charts while I continued to walk. We talked about my condition and he told me that because of my stenosis, I could really jeopardize my health if I fell on my back, neck, or head. He added that running should be okay. If I fell forward I could brace the fall and soften the impact with my hands. We talked about a young foolish man who was again in the hospital as a result of a skiing accident. "You don't want to end up like him; he doesn't seem to get it," was the doctor's comment. Brain and traumatic injury are very common among that age group. This physician then told me that all they were doing for me was essentially just the neck brace. He went on to say, "You don't need to be here; you can take meds at home. The brace is to be worn all the time and I mean all the time." I was just excited I could leave!

I called Linda at home. She had planned to return to the hospital early that afternoon, but I changed her plans. I excitedly said, "Come and pick me up!" She replied, "What are you talking about? Last time I saw you, you were barfing. I don't believe you." I quickly responded with, "I don't care. Come pick me up. Talk to the nurse if you like but pick me up." I started to get ready so I could leave my little entrapment. Linda arrived, and we said our goodbyes to all the staff. Linda drove to the drugstore to pick up my prescriptions, but I had decided to only take over-the-counter meds. Who needs to be on heavy, numbing, prescription medication? I didn't want any part of that.

Super Bowl Sunday arrived after a miserable sleepless Saturday night. I belonged to a Monday night football group and that year Linda and I were again the Super Bowl hosts. However, my role that year involved just sitting in a chair. I discovered that a rocking chair with a high back worked the best. I was on over-the-counter meds and was told to watch how I walked. They didn't want me tripping on rugs or things like that. In addition to my neck brace, I also sported a huge red-colored hematoma on my forehead.

From what I remember of the accident, my head landed between Gypsy's front legs. What a great mare, she didn't move even an inch. Linda carefully led her away from me, and tied both Gypsy and Raider to a tree some distance down the trail. There was speculation that I hit my head first before the rest of my body landed on terra firma. The rest of Sunday was spent with people at the house, the Super Bowl game, and my telling of the story.

I had a doctor's appointment scheduled with the orthopedic surgeon in three weeks. Every day and especially each night were difficult for me. I was extremely uncomfortable during this miserable period of my life. However, I made one major life-changing decision; I was through with competitive riding. This meant that I did not intend to compete in Ride & Tie or endurance events. For me the rush was riding a galloping horse. I don't enjoy just sitting on the horse, nor did I get a thrill riding on a walking or trotting horse. I was now terrified of having a horse accident. I simply did not want to end up paralyzed. Accidents happen to riders on horseback all the time. I knew plenty of people who had been seriously injured by falling off their horses. Keep in mind that these individuals are experienced and good riders. I did not want to chance my horse stumbling or tripping and me getting injured. At this point, I did not have a plan for Gypsy or Raider.

I realized quickly that I couldn't tolerate sitting, or not being able to perform simple things like washing my face or taking a shower. Being incapacitated was definitely not my style. If I couldn't be active, I was likely to get seriously depressed. Even though I received counsel from

Linda and Jonathan to re-think my decision about never competing in Ride & Tie and endurance, I remained firm with my decision.

This was going to be a major change in my lifestyle. What was a life without horses? Now, with all this idle time, I began thinking about writing a book. I'm certain that having this time available greatly influenced my decision. I don't know if I would have told my story if the accident had not happened.

Linda drove me to the hospital to meet the surgeon for my three-week appointment. I had not seen this physician since my stay in the hospital. First there were X-rays. Rod, the head of the X-ray department and a former Ride & Tie person, was in charge. I first met him a number of years before on the Wednesday evening trail run that takes place at the Overlook in Auburn. We talked while my X-rays were embedded on film, and then I was to see the doctor. I first talked with the nurse, and she mentioned that patients are usually in a neck brace for about six weeks. We discussed all the do's and don'ts of this whole routine, and she told me most of the information that I wanted answered. I met with the doctor and he announced that I didn't have to wear that uncomfortable neck brace anymore. At first, I didn't believe what I was hearing as my mind was preparing to wear this brace for another three to six weeks. I was flabbergasted! After asking him to repeat his liberating proclamation, the doctor directed me to gradually remove the brace. I wasn't cleared to run since he was still concerned about the jarring issue from running down the trail. The numbness and tingling sensations in my fingers were becoming less and less and I knew that I was improving. My bones were healing and the doctor wanted to see me again in six weeks.

I began to walk the trails and although I could see where I was going, I was still worried about tripping. I was unsure of my stability, and really afraid of falling on my face. My mood was markedly better, as was my energy. I was better. What a relief to feel more normal and able to spend more time outdoors. Being in a wonderful outdoor environment always brought peace and serenity to my life. The role of the environment and its importance quickly became very clear to me.

Six weeks later, I arrived for the next doctor's appointment. I again had X-rays, talked to the nurse, and met with the doctor. He reported, "The bones are healing nicely." He suggested that because of my stenosis condition, I could have surgery to make me symptom-free. There are all sorts of complications that happen when the spinal cord pinches on various nerves. Loss of balance and encopresis are just a few of the problems that can occur. I talked about recovery, rehabilitation, and concluded that I wanted nothing to do with an operation. The doctor admitted that there was nothing more he could do for me and released me from his care. I was now cleared, which meant I could hit the trail again and resume my running addiction. Good news, in fact it was the best news I had heard in nine weeks.

I began research on the doctor's plate procedure and my stenosis condition. I talked to my sister who helped me by researching stenosis on the Internet. I talked with my brother and he claimed, among other things, that surgeries are not always the right thing to do. My cousin through marriage has a sister who is married to neurologist, Norm Rotter. Incidentally, Norm is the neurologist who evaluated my brother Ron when he fell off the porch and hit his head while in high school. To add to that "six degrees of separation," my first wife and I looked at a duplex that Norm and his wife Harriet were selling on West Outer Drive in Detroit; it's a small world. My cousin Richard Komer married Judy, Harriet's younger sister. I called Judy, told her the story about my accident, and conveyed that I wanted to talk with Norm.

Norm called and we discussed the series of events and various options. He asked if I had lateral X-rays taken. I told him that I didn't know. He asked that I send the records to him in care of the Department of Neurology, Henry Ford Hospital. Thanks to his advice, I had another X-ray, and after Norm assessed it he reassured me and confirmed the fact that I was stable. We talked about prognosis, surgery, and my lifestyle. It was clear to me that there would be no surgery at this time.

Now I could focus on my running. I had to recondition my muscles, tendons, ligaments and lungs; improve my cardio; and do my heat training. I began to increase my running distance to 20-plus miles, and one hot day I ran from my house to Cool and back. I decided to run (okay, walk) up Maine Bar, which is about a mile long with lots of elevation, which means it's a long, big, steep, and difficult climb. It's part of the Way Too Cool run. Everything was going hunky-dory until I started my climb. As a rule, I was able to walk and run up the trail without stopping. Let me emphasize that I walked most of the way. The trail was steep, rocky, and full of ruts. I had to stop; I was just unable to continue as I was having trouble breathing. I continued to walk a little bit and then stopped in an attempt to catch my breath. I then became concerned and thought I may have been experiencing arterial fibrillation. I finally returned home after quite a struggle. I was exhausted, whipped, and simply worn out. I made an appointment with Dr. Hook. I wanted to get an EKG to evaluate my heart. The EKG read normal; I believe I simply didn't have enough heat training for that climb. That meant I still wasn't in great running condition. I must admit being relieved, knowing that I was okay and just needed more training in the heat. As you might suspect, I wasn't done competing.

A friend, Sue Smyth, told me about a run at Salt Point. A bunch of Ride & Tie people I knew, including Sue were planning on running. On Friday, Linda and I drove to Salt Point from Marin County along Highway One. The drive was magnificent, with the Pacific Ocean to the west and the mountains to the east. We eventually reached the Vaughn Homestead, which consisted of two rustic cabins surrounded by a magnificent view of the ocean and its geological treasure of rock formations.

We all left for the starting line on Saturday morning. The 50K race began in the fog on a plot of land adjacent to the ocean. Then the three race loops headed into the mountains and inland where it was stifling hot. I felt good for the first two loops and then decided to take it easy on the third loop because of some discomfort, especially on the downhill. I finished and was very pleased with myself. This was a good first test for me. I handled the distance pretty well on my first competitive race since my accident.

Jack Sholl and I developed a great rapport, and he helped spark an interest in me for rowing in a one-person shell (sculling). Linda and I ended up taking sculling lessons at the aquatic center at Folsom Lake. Jack referred us to Bob Whitford, the administrator and former rowing coach. I discovered that Bob's brother was an outrigger canoe coach in Southern California. And to make things more interesting, he coached Linda's two daughters Kristie and Sidne. Now I had an entrée into water sports. This was exciting, and I owe this newly-found enthusiasm to Jack. At the aquatic center, aside from sculling in the water, they had a top-notch workout facility including the Concept 2 rowing machine. Linda and I started working out there but unfortunately, Linda developed sciatica (a problem in her buttocks) that plagued her for a while.

My next running race, the Helen Klein Race, was at the end of October. I entered the 50-mile event and asked Tony Brickel, Sue Smyth, and Steve Anderson to be my pacers. Steve began pacing me after about 10 miles, and ran approximately 20 miles with me. The first 25 miles were okay, but at about 35 miles I began to hurt. I could not run without pain. I could walk fast, though. Tony walked with me and I began to get concerned about making the cut-off time. I finally took some Advil and was able to run again. Sue paced me the last five to eight miles until we got to the finish. I just barely made the 12-hour cut-off. I was happy that I was able to complete this difficult run. It was Halloween so I said to Linda, "Let's go home and dress up for the parties tonight."

XIV

Jack Sholl: Patriot, Rower, Gentleman Unparalleled

Jack Sholl, born October 30, 1925, is one of rowing's most respected and revered legends. And in his mid 80s, Jack still continues to compete in rowing. Jack has been competing for 64 years in this sport at all age levels.

Jack also defines himself as a patriot. He's a proud member of the Sons of the American Revolution and has served as president of the Coachella Valley chapter. It's interesting to note that Jack's grandfather Peter Shumaker met William Penn eight generations ago. Yes, the William Penn who was a champion of democracy and religious freedom as well as the founder of the Province of Pennsylvania. The principles he established for the Pennsylvania Government served as an inspiration for the U.S. Constitution. Jack's grandfather met Penn along with a group of farmers in the late 1600s in Germany. Penn encouraged them to come to the 'new land,' and Peter Shumaker did just that in 1695. Another relative of Jack's owned a tavern near Philadelphia, and to Jack's surprise he learned that this relative played a significant role in the Underground Railroad, a network of persons who helped escaped slaves on their way to freedom in the northern states in the 1800s.

A few years ago, Jack was scheduled to be a guest speaker for two Sons of the American Revolution presentations at Independence Hall in Philadelphia. Even though he was in pain and was taking painkillers because of his multiple myeloma (cancer of the bone marrow), he still arrived to give his presentations. He quipped, "I didn't want to walk in with the aid of a cane, but I did so in spite of my vanity." After the first presentation, Jack was invited to lunch by the committee. They planned to visit a tavern that, according to history, was a favorite drinking and eating spot of none other than John Adams. Jack sadly declined because of his physical discomfort. He added, "I wanted to go but I was hurting too much. But I received good feedback about my presentations; they liked them."

Jack frequently gives historical presentations all over the country. In my discussion with Jack, he didn't think I knew about Hyam Solomon. I told him I had learned about Hyam and the fact that he helped finance the American Revolutionary War. Jack responded with, "I frequently give PowerPoint presentations about George Washington going to Hyam for financial support for the war effort. Hyam did not let Washington down. He was able to get contributions from his synagogue to support the Revolutionary War; he was a real patriot."

Jack also contributes time as a volunteer for the U.S. Coast Guard in San Diego, California. He is very proud to be associated with those who keep this country safe.

Jack volunteers for the National Park Service in Philadelphia. Each summer he conducts half-hour tours of the West Wing in Independence Hall at the Independence National Historical Park. He's a prolific reader of American history, with emphasis on the presidents. Jack ends his tours reminding people that Philadelphia is the birthplace of America. After his presentations people frequently ask him, "Did you teach American history in high school or in college?" His consistent answer is, "No, I worked for IBM for 29 years."

Jack tells an engaging story that incorporated his experience as a volunteer at Independence Hall and his identity as a patriot. In February 2004, he was stationed as a volunteer at the actual Liberty Bell. Several well-dressed gentleman approached him and asked if they were permitted to take his picture in front of the Bell. After they snapped the photograph, they mentioned it was likely to wind up in a glossy brochure distributed throughout France. These men told Jack that with the permission of the National Park Service, they had scientifically copied the Liberty Bell dimensions the previous night. They added, "We are going to cast an exact replica for our bell, of course without the crack that would ring in E flat." This glossy brochure was to advertise their "Normandy Liberty Bell," to be unveiled in May 2004. They hoped to get permission to install it in the American Military Cemetery at Omaha Beach in Normandy.

Jack asked these gentlemen if they would like to participate in a Fourth of July ceremony called "Let Freedom Ring." This ceremony was directed by an act of Congress which states that the U.S. Liberty Bell is to be tapped 13 times by direct descendents of the signers of the Declaration of Independence at exactly 2:00 p.m. Philadelphia time. Jack was not a ringing member of that ceremony, but he helped recruit over 13,000 bells to be rung at the appointed hour. Churches, school-houses, Army bases, city halls, etc., participated in the ceremony. Jack asked his new French friends if they would ring the Normandy Liberty Bell 13 times on the Fourth of July at 8:00 p.m. Normandy time. They agreed.

In 2004 Jack attended an international rowing championship Regatta for master oarsmen in Hamburg, Germany. After the competition, Jack drove to Normandy where he met with Patrick Daudon, the man responsible for casting the Normandy Liberty Bell. Jack asked Daudon if the Normandy Bell could be sent to Philadelphia for the July 4, 2005 "Let Freedom Ring" ceremony. Jack used his influence as a member of the Pennsylvania Society of Sons of the American Revolution to get the Pentagon involved with the project. Governmental wheels turned, and the U.S. Navy delivered the Normandy Bell to Philadelphia for the celebration.

A few days before the Fourth of July, the Philadelphia Inquirer published an article about Jack and the Normandy Liberty Bell. The reporter asked if Jack was going to be one of the bell ringers that year, to which Jack replied "No." Shortly after the story was published, numerous readers contacted the Inquirer suggesting that Jack should be a bell ringer. That did it! Jack rang the bell with great pride. He told me, "It was one of the greatest thrills of my life and it all happened by fate."

In 1942, Jack was a junior in high school and wanted to enlist in the service in order to protect his country. At that time, enlistment required parental consent. His parents weren't willing to sign the mandatory papers, so a rebellious Jack left high school immediately and went to work as a ship fitter apprentice on the USS Wisconsin.

At the shipyard, boxing was the main source of entertainment for the men during lunchtime. Each fight lasted three rounds or less. At the time Jack weighed 145 pounds. He won his very first fight. In his second fight, he fought a heavyweight. That lunchtime fight, my friends, was his last. But do not get the impression that Jack wasn't tough. He was (and is) plenty tough . . .

As a boy of about 10, Jack got into a fistfight with a neighborhood bully who bloodied Jack's nose during the fight. Jack returned home with blood spattered on his face, whereupon his father took a good look at him and became angry with Jack, so it seemed. His father immediately and I mean immediately, marched Jack back to the bully's house. Jack fought him again but this time he bloodied the bully's nose. That was the last time that bully ever picked on Jack.

When Jack was asked what lessons he learned from his father, Jack proudly replied, "To stand up for your rights, don't back down, and do not quit." Jack learned that early lesson well, and it continued to guide him. Jack does not know how to quit.

After spending that year at the shipyards, he did join the service and fought honorably for his country.

Jack attributes parental support for some of his success. His father paid for trumpet lessons when he was a kid, as well as the Boy Scout paraphernalia he needed. His parents came to his functions and always told him he did a great job. He still remembers his mother bragging to others about him. Jack does well with extrinsic reinforcement. External praise is one of his motivators.

After returning home from the service in 1946, Jack attended a Philadelphia Phillies baseball game with a buddy. Upon finding his stadium seat, an attractive young female usher appeared and dusted off the seat. He thought to himself, "She's cute" (and probably more that he didn't tell me). She returned later on in the game and asked Jack if he would meet her at the Pennsylvania Athletic Club. Not being shy, coupled with the fact that usher Rita Lyons was pretty, he quickly said,

"Yes." Jack joined her at the club, the very club, in fact, where he was introduced to rowing; a sport he has excelled in for over 64 years.

That meeting with Rita changed the direction of Jack's future. Upon returning from the service, he simply didn't know what path to take in life. His father put pressure on him to go into the trades. He wondered what to do.

While rowing for the Pennsylvania Athletic Club, Jack's coach Rusty Callow told him that he could help Jack get admitted to the University of Washington. Jack took him up on the offer, and was welcomed at the college in 1948 where he eventually graduated in 1953. Jack also rowed for the University of Washington while studying there.

In 1950, Jack literally met his wife Joan on the Schuylkill River. Joan was rowing down the river while Jack was rowing in the opposite direction. Never shy, Jack managed to find Joan, and ultimately courted and married her. Joan was a member of the only girls rowing club at that time.

Jack and Joan had two sons. To no one's surprise, one son rowed for the University of Washington and the other son rowed for the University of California at Berkeley. To further bolster the family's ties to rowing, Joan was the first woman Olympic official in rowing, officiating at the Games in Atlanta, Georgia in 1984.

After graduating from college in 1953, Jack returned to Philadelphia and went to work for John B. Kelly, the Olympian rower. When I was talking to Jack about this part of his life, he casually mentioned that John B. Kelly was Grace Kelly's father. According to Jack, Franklin D. Roosevelt supposedly said, "John Kelly is the most handsome man I've ever met." Jack, of course, was also introduced to Grace Kelly's husband, Prince Rainier. Not only was he a patriot, Jack also associated with royalty.

In 1955 Jack joined IBM. He was on the ground floor of the computer world, and stayed with IBM for 29 years. He moved to New Jersey, New York, Pennsylvania, and finally to California in 1981. He was the ultimate company man, working long hours to climb his way up the corporate ladder. He traveled all over the world, and trained many of the CEOs of large corporations about computers. Even though he gave his all to the company, he still found time to jog during the week and row on weekends. In those days, the company always came first. Jack eventually retired in 1996 at the age of 71.

I asked Jack to describe his favorite race. He told me his most memorable rowing race took place in Strathclyde, Scotland in 1988 at the World's Masters Regatta. His crew averaged 60 years of age. In the first lane was the USA with Jack's boat. On the port side in Lane 2 was the German crew. Jack remembers that each member of the German crew was a veteran of World War II. And every member of the USA crew was a veteran of World War II. Jack's crew never discussed this openly. His emotions were at a high level, much more so than his normal pre-race jitters. At the command "row!" the USA boat was off to a good start. The Germans also started well. Twenty strokes into the race, the other four crews quickly fell behind the front runners. Now the Americans and Germans were neck and neck. With each stroke, the crews struggled to get ahead while searching for a psychological advantage. Both coxswains were yelling commands and encouragement as loudly as possible. The German coxswain, being the loudest, influenced one of Jack's crewmembers. He later told Jack that he started to take his cadence from the German.

The two crews did not yield, and because of the overwhelming roar of the spectators on shore, it was difficult to hear the voice of the U.S. coxswain. At the last 500-meter mark, the two crews were still even. At about the 300-meter mark, Jack's body wanted to quit. He didn't want to take one more stroke. The coxswain yelled, "Thirty more! Don't let the Germans beat you!" Jack's buddy and bowman, Gus Constant, shouted, "You and me Jack, you and me!" Jack said it psyched him when he heard Gus. Inwardly, Jack immediately called himself a "coward." Jack told me he pulled as hard as he could, thinking, "I've got a gold medal; just don't quit. One more stroke, one more stroke, and then one more stroke."

The Germans didn't quit. Jack was looking frantically for the finish line. Then he heard two sharp blasts from an air gun. The race was over, and all the rowers slumped over their oars. Jack didn't even know if the first blast was for the U.S. or for the German crew. In suspense, they waited for the official announcement. The announcer finally said, "Etas Unis to the awards dock." What a relief! What joy! The USA was the winner by 49/100 of a second.

In 2005 in Strathclyde, Scotland, Jack met a German crew member from the 1988 race. The German revealed that, "I still row that race mentally many times," referring to the 1988 competition. Jack added, "It was my most memorable race also."

I asked Jack how he accomplishes all that he does, what his secrets are, and what his "self-talk" is all about. He stated, "I never consider that I age. My attitude is always that of a young person, and my physical appearance belies my age. In fact, I believe retirement is the greatest indignity thrust upon humanity. Even now, at age 85, I want to stay active. In fact, psychologically I think of myself as a 40-year-old. I feel great, and I hope to row deep into my 80s. I have aspirations of reaching 90. It is critical that I set goals and try to achieve them. This forces me to stay in top physical condition. Otherwise, I am likely to become a couch potato."

It's apparent that goal setting and thinking about the future are significant parts of how Jack operates. This is simply the way he is. He continues to develop his mind and his body. He is a positive thinker. In the year 2010, he was unable to participate in the world championship because of bone marrow cancer. However, he recently said with a glint in his eye, "I have high hopes of being on the port side of an eight-oared crew in Poznan, Poland in September of 2011."

Jack employs the following "self-talk" when struggling during an event. "I can't quit, I'll take one more stroke," and "I can't let the crew down." And when it really gets bad: "I am a coward, I'm quitting," and "I'm not going to row anymore." This helps his self-motivation. He even thinks, "Maybe the others will quit." So Jack, like everyone else, struggles during difficult times. However, he uses his thinking to push himself. Notice that he uses both positive and negative thinking. He uses his negative thoughts as motivation and then turns them into a positive. He's obviously been very successful with this method.

More insight into Jack's character is illustrated when he talks about his comrades dealing with pain. For Jack, competitive rowers embrace severe pain as an ally. Extremely motivated, they routinely push through pain thresholds not routinely encountered. They live in a world where pain is exhorted on the tee shirts they wear (pain is weakness leaving the body, no pain no gain, I am not afraid of the pain, if you could see the pain it would blind you, pain means progress, bring it on, character cannot be developed without pain). Agonies in rowing are synonymous terms.

Jack's positive thinking, goal setting, and competitive nature are a big part of his triumphant story. How does this 85-year-old competitive man continue to row? This man has won 19 international Masters Crew races between 1985 and 2006 in both four and eight man crews, with and without coxswain. He has won 15 U.S. national gold medals. In 2009, at an international competition held in Vienna, Jack was a member of a crew that had an average age of 80. He wanted to be the first crew to win a gold medal in that age bracket and did so.

One might wonder how this 85-year-old man retains the skills necessary to row. Anyone who has been in a shell realizes the required level of difficulty. I know, because I have been at Lake Natoma in a one man shell. The shell is long, narrow, and designed to go in one direction straight ahead. Just watch a rower get into a shell and marvel at the required technique. This means hang on to the two oars or you're likely to wind up in the water as I did. It takes strength, grit, and technique. Jack has all three.

Jack's reasons for competing include, "It's an ego thing. I can't disappoint others or let them down. Even though I say this is my last year, I've been saying that every year for the last few years. I realize I like the competition, I like the affiliation, and the bonding with others my age. It's been a way of life for me. I want to live life to its fullest and I might be afraid to stop, afraid to retire."

It's clear that setting expectations and attaining goals are driving forces for Jack. Because competitions are so encompassing for him, it becomes who he is. It is his self. His complex identity is comprised of being both a patriot and a rower.

XV

Ms. Outrigger Doc Shay: The Quintessential Athlete

Linda and I took a trip to the Big Island of Hawaii to vacation and to meet with Sharon "Shay" Bintliff, known to the world simply as "Doc Shay." We spent a few days in Waimea, where I ran along the highway to get my running fix, which is so critical for my well-being. We were told about a great swimming location and we took advantage of that super spot. After our stay in Waimea, we ventured towards Hilo. We had dinner at the observatory at the University of Hawaii and then made our way to the volcano house.

That evening we made contact with Gino Ortez, a friend of Linda's, and arranged to meet him and his boys the following afternoon. Gino is a character, to say the least. He shares his remarkable knowledge of the role of muscles in the body with students at his massage therapy school in Kona. In fact, because of Linda's injury, he used her for a demonstration for his class. Gino told great stories about his two Olympic medical experiences, one in Los Angeles and the other in Salt Lake.

We toured one of the Big Island's five volcanoes, where Gino's sons were the tour guides. We spent our evenings at the black sand beach and had the pleasure of meeting Gino's friends. I talked with him about my running and was even thinking that he'd be a great trainer. He suggested that I read about plyometrics and he referred me to Bob Anderson's book, "Stretching." I started to incorporate information Gino had suggested, and we talked about putting a race on at the Big Island.

Our next stay was on the large, sheltered natural bay of Captain Cook for one evening, and then on to Kona. Every time, and I mean every time I go to Hawaii, I get so excited about the possibility of living there. It's a fantasy of mine to live on the islands.

The Super Bowl of paddling takes place in Hawaii, where outrigger canoes race from the island of Molokai to the island of Oahu. This race is the oldest and most prestigious outrigger race in the world. The paddlers have to navigate and cross one of the roughest inner island channels in existence, simulating the ancient Polynesians method of water travel. Ocean conditions can vary from calm as a lake, to turbulent; competitors can be faced with extreme winds and huge waves. Coastal currants and tide factors from Oahu also play a significant part in how this race is executed. In other words, there is potential constant chaos. This event is a test of preparation, endurance, strength and paddling prowess. For those with Hawaiian roots, this event is a "crossing," not simply a race. Channel conditions influence the choice of route the canoes take between the two islands. The distance of the races has varied from 38.66 to 42 miles. If that's not enough, the steersmen do not always take the most direct route.

A paddler by the name of "Toots" Minvielle was born on the island of Oahu on June 1, 1903. He attained a degree in engineering and surveying from the University of Hawaii. Minvielle was a member of the local Outrigger Canoe Club since 1917. He knew that the ancient Polynesians traveled between the islands by outrigger canoe, and Minvielle had a dream to continue the tradition. He began discussing the possibility of staging a crossing of outrigger canoes between the two islands and elevating it to a race. The time was 1949, after World War II. His idea was not well received by the board of his Canoe Club, but this did not dissuade him from pursuing it. Feedback varied from, "It's too dangerous" and "it's too far," to "there are too many logistical problems." The U.S. Coast Guard also attempted to stop him from putting on the race.

Finally, in 1952, the first outrigger race from Molokai to Oahu began with three canoes. Their finishing times ranged from 8 hours and 55 minutes to 9 hours and 13 minutes. Reflective of that era, the participants in the Outrigger canoes were all of male gender. A group of women paddlers in 1954 lobbied the men to become part of the race, but were turned down. The men's race was called the Molokai Hoe.

Women paddlers continued to build a groundswell campaign for participating in this crossing from Molokai to Oahu. The U.S. Coast Guard heard about this campaign. It's too dangerous, no place for women, it's too rough, etc. was their general attitude. These determined women rallied, and on October 12, 1975, the Healani Canoe Club launched the first women crossing. Unofficially, they put on their own race from Molokai to Oahu for two outrigger canoes. The other canoe was an all-star crew made up of women from several other canoe clubs. The winning race time by the Healani women was 7 hours 15 minutes. They accomplished all this without the blessing of the canoe association.

On October 14, 1979, these women finally held their first official race that covered 40.8 miles. The rules of the race were similar to the men's regulations, but differed in that each team was allowed 12 paddlers, 6 in the canoe and 6 in the escort boats. The men had a total of 9 paddlers. In that 1979 crossing there were 17 canoes and all the teams finished. The winning crew was from the Outrigger Canoe Club and their time was 6 hours and 35 minutes. This race was called the Na Wahineo Ke Kai. So to this day, women have a race of their own that takes place a few weeks before the men's race.

Sharon "Shay" Bintliff was on one of the two outrigger canoes in the 1975 maiden voyage. Remarkably, she has continued to race across the dangerous channel every year since then, even in 2009 in the Senior Masters Division at the age of 74. She is the oldest female to ever compete in this event and made her 30th crossing in 2009. This woman is known as "Doc Shay" and her name is a story too.

Her mother liked the name Sharon, which is on her birth certificate. However, her grandmother loved the name Shay, and that is what she is called. The moniker "Doc" was earned when she claimed her medical degree. Her medical specialty is pediatrics and EMR, a job even tougher than outrigger canoe racing.

Shay was born on September 5, 1935 in Longview, Texas. When I met her, I found Doc Shay to be intelligent, outgoing, and full of life, although she believed that she didn't fit in while growing up in

Texas. She wasn't quiet and demure as many other young women, rather she was athletic, active and could hold her own with the boys. She described her mother as being very athletic, by virtue of the fact that she sang and danced in vaudeville. She even included Shay onstage at the age of three. Shay likes to please, and she also liked the reinforcement received when performing with her mother and she still likes the reinforcement she receives when competing. Growing up, she loved the water and was terrific at golf. You name the sport, and she can do it.

Shay was her nickname growing up from elementary through high school. While attending college and medical school, she went by her birth name of Sharon. She went back to using Shay while working as an intern at Highland Hospital in Oakland, California, and has used Shay ever since.

In Shay's high school days, the girls didn't have a golf team. Shay practiced with the boys, who had their own team. It didn't take long for everyone to realize that Shay was the better golfer. She believed that her mother was a positive influence on her being competitive. It also didn't hurt to have a father who competed in baseball, football, and golf.

In high school Shay was on the tennis team, but she was too short for volleyball. She concentrated on golf. She played golf with her neighbor who happened to be the local golf pro at the country club. His assessment of Shay's talent was, "This little midget has a natural swing." This golf pro, Jack Smith, encouraged her and gave her positive reinforcement. It also helped that she drove the ball really well and played a smart game. She won the women's amateur golf tournament in Texas, and teamed up with Patty Berg in an LPGA pro-am golf competition. She recalled pro-Patty saying, "Are you going to join the LPGA tour?" She replied, "No, I'm going to medical school." Patty responded, "Good, Shay, you become a doctor and every Wednesday afternoon take your doctor friends out on the golf course and clean their clocks!" And she did just that. Recently, the senior golf pro Fuzzy Zoeller said after Shay hit her long drive, "It's little Wie!" referring to the female golf pro Michelle Wie.

Doc Shay began medical school at the University of Texas at Galveston. She married and then transferred to the University of Washington to complete her medical school training. At that time, in 1962, she was the only female in the medical program of 76 students. Her interest was in pediatrics, and upon graduation, she had two offers. One position was in Vermont and the second was at the University of Hawaii medical school on the island of Oahu. Since she grew up on the Gulf Coast at Galveston, the decision was easy. She was at peace with the ocean, and considered herself a water person. In 1965, Shay, her husband and two children moved to Oahu, and she began developing the Birth Defects Center at the University of Hawaii.

Doc Shay was interested in pediatrics, birth defects, and genetics. She was influenced by her teacher and mentor Dr. David Smith while in training at the University of Washington. She had given birth to her second son, and after graduation she took off six months to be with her two boys. Dr. Smith arranged for her to have a fellowship in birth defects. He knew that it was important for Shay to raise her boys and spend time with them, so he did the unheard of by allowing her to complete a one-year program over a period of two years.

What impressed Shay was that Dr. Smith was interested in causes of birth defects, and problems related to subsequent births by the mother. She was also impressed that he was interested in helping the child develop his potential within the family unit. Back then, there weren't many tests available to assist in the assessment and diagnosis for these special children. Chromosomal studies were just becoming available. This training was invaluable to her. The University of Hawaii position was a perfect fit. She was given free reign by the Pediatric Department at the University of Hawaii Medical School to develop the first birth defects department within pediatrics.

From 1965 through 1982, Doc Shay was in charge of the Birth Defects Center at the University of Hawaii. Even though it was challenging, this position was not enough for her and she took on a second job. She became the medical director of the Waimano Home for Children and Adults with Developmental Delay. In this residential setting, she took advantage of the opportunity to set up a training program for University of Hawaii medical students. The training program was to give these future doctors various types of experiences with patients who had developmental disabilities diagnoses.

Her training program helped these students by giving them practical and pedantic experience to help them diagnose these individuals. They received first-hand experience observing the patients live and play in a non–clinical environment. Shay indicated that she had learned so much about, and from these individuals. She was amazed by the way these people were able to overcome their disabilities and achieve at the levels that they did.

How did this professional woman, with two boys and a husband, find the time to bike, run, paddle, ride, surf, compete in triathlons, and run a marathon? Shay said that the biking part was easy, because she lived on the top of a mountain road in Oahu. While working at the University of Hawaii, she would ride down the hill to work and ride up the hill to return home; a smart way for her to use this environmentally sound mode of transportation and train at the same time.

Shay's involvement in paddling was the result of volunteering her time as a medical doctor in her boys' sports activities. By volunteering, she got to know and meet the other boys' parents, some of whom were members of the Healani Canoe Club. So, in the 1970s she started paddling in outrigger canoe races. She's athletic, loves the ocean, and likes to swim. Paddling became a natural for her. She is also persistent, manages her time well, looks to the future, and is goal directed.

Doc Shay believes that she was influenced in becoming a doctor partially as result of painful and excruciating ear infections as a child. The doctor who treated her, Dr. Engeldow, used ether as an anesthetic and then lanced her ears. When she woke up after the procedure, she was without pain. She stated, "I was immediately interested in being a doctor. I thought that whole procedure was a miracle."

In 1969, she visited the Big Island of Hawaii with her two sons, their Labrador Retriever, and Shay's mother. Shay rented a camper and they explored the entire island, visiting the blackened sand beaches as well as the military camp at the volcano summit. One goal was to show her mom an active volcano. They took various hiking and side trips, visiting the many steam vents at the volcano summit. About nine o'clock one evening, there was a knock on the camper. She opened the door and there stood a park ranger, who said, "I suggest visiting the Pu'oosteam vent right now, because Madam Pele is blowing!" So they took off to find Pele, the Goddess of Volcanoes. When they arrived at the steam vent, she handed her mother the binoculars. When Shay's mother saw the volcano Kilauea erupting about 300 feet in the air, she yelled, "Holy shit!" in her deep Texas drawl. The adjoining crowd enjoyed a good laugh.

In the 1970s, Doc Shay's outrigger paddling buddies, a group of young females, decided to start a women's soccer league in Honolulu. They wanted to stay in good shape during the paddling off-season. Most of these younger women were from Tahiti and were excellent soccer players. Doc Shay was older and in her mid 40s. She was a marathon runner, believed she could run with these youngsters, and was so excited to think that she could learn to play soccer too. She knew these young team members were somewhat skeptical about her being able to keep up with them. But she was determined to do well. She noticed that when they had a very hard practice or would run wind sprints, they would ask her "Hey, Doc, are you okay?" After a while she began to get annoyed. Well, one day the team was running wind sprints, and after quite a few she remembers bending over trying to catch her breath. Then she saw lying on the ground one of those small, round batteries that is found in watches. She picked it up, stood straight up and in a loud voice hollered, "Oh shit!" Several of her teammates immediately responded with, "Doc, are you okay? What's wrong?" She then held up the battery and proclaimed, "Oh no! The battery just fell out of my pacemaker!" Shay continues, "Well, the look on my teammates' faces was sheer panic. I could not keep a straight face, and I started laughing. When they realized what I had done, they got mad. They poured ice water on me and tried to take off all my clothes and started throwing soccer balls at me. Then we were all laughing! That was truly a memory never to be forgotten." This episode is a good insight into Doc Shay's playful character.

Anne Perry has been Doc Shay's friend for about 30 years. Anne described Doc Shay as a team player who was very generous with her time and money. Anne stated that Shay is a wonderful mentor because she's involved in such a variety of things, and was even given the YWCA women's leadership award one year. She volunteers her time as a doctor at the Ironman events on the Big Island and does the same with the double Ironman competition.

At the age of 48, Doc Shay went back to school to train to become an emergency room doctor. She's a good mother and a very good role model for women in medicine and sports. She's always available and gives back to others. Anne recalled that one time her mother collapsed and was taken to the hospital, and Doc Shay came to visit. Doc Shay has won numerous awards, and you could write a book on just her achievements. She even drives young golfers crazy with her game, because she plays it so smartly.

Dr. Tony Giassoli met Doc Shay about 16 years ago in the emergency room at the Honokoa Hospital on the Big Island of Hawaii where she was the medical director. Dr. Giassoli was just out of his residency and had arrived there from El Paso, Texas. He said, "She was a good mentor and helped me tremendously. Personally, she's quite compassionate towards patients and feels very strongly about spousal abuse. She always asked her patients, is it safe at home? She is funny and always has a joke to share with staff and patients alike. She makes kids feel safe and has a good bedside manner. She collects medical supplies that we throw away and sends them to a clinic in India."

In the past, when not competing in outrigger canoe races, Doc Shay would spend her off season time playing soccer and competing in triathlons. She is no longer able to run, so now her off-season training consists of swimming, biking, working out on a rowing machine, and paddling in her single canoe. As far as swimming goes, she swims in a small bay that is about 100 yards wide. Next to the bay, golfers tee off from the third hole at the Mauna Kea Golf Course. If they hit the ball well, their ball won't fall into the ocean; those not so lucky send their golf balls plopping into the small bay. Doc Shay swims back and forth in the channel and free-dives to pick up the errant balls. "I have a collection of balls from all the great golf settings in the world," Doc Shay smiles.

She does this 'exercise' at least once a week and finds the ocean mentally and spiritually uplifting. She may bike for an hour two times a week and row on her rowing machine for 30 minutes once a week, working up a sweat and raising her pulse to over 100. She also paddles in the ocean in her single canoe once a week; her fun activities are always varied. Her regatta racing schedule begins in May and ends in August, and the long distance races begin in August and go through the end of September.

When I asked Doc Shay to share some of her secrets about her extraordinary life, she stated, "You have to believe in yourself and not what others say about you, like you're too little or you're a female so you can't do it." Any kind of negative input or feedback resulted in her saying to herself, "Yes, you can." Shay added that her best teacher was her mother.

Shay continued to reflect, saying, "I also learned not to let my ego get in the way of purpose. If you have a mission to do something, you can't place your ego over the mission." She gave an example of a March of Dimes fund raising event. "They wanted to have a party honoring me in an attempt to bring in more people because they knew me. They thought that by doing that they would raise more money. I insisted that the people on the frontlines, the people volunteering their time and energy, are the ones who should be honored and get the recognition. The goal was to raise money, not for me to be in the newspaper."

Her philosophy in life is like the Kevin Spacey movie, "Pay It Forward." In that movie, the theme was to get three others to do good deeds, and then those three would also each get three others to do the same. Thus you have a ripple effect of people doing good deeds by giving to others, and getting others to do likewise. Shay's tombstone might read, "To Be Continued." In other words, "You can't get rid of me."

Sammie Stanbro, age 65, is Shay's fellow paddler and competitor. She called Doc a legend. Her comments were, "Shay has great perseverance, and nothing, no nothing, ever stops her. She always has a joke to tell, is compassionate about her animals, and she is game for anything. She's always active. She's great. And she's a doctor, so you can ask her for medical information and she will oblige you with ways to fix things. During one event, she was bloody, but she was oblivious to the blood. It was clear that her focus was on the canoe and not about her injury. You will learn from her that, 'You don't give up.' I would much rather have her on my team, than have to compete against her!"

One of Dr. Bintliff's favorite memories is, in her own words: "I am blessed with so many memories of the Molokai to Oahu Na Wahine canoe race. There is one that always will be ever present and at the top of the list, the special gift of the Palaoa I received from Mitchell Pauoili, the Honorable Mayor of Molokai. I first met Mitchell in the late 1960s when I started conducting neighbor island Birth Defects Clinics. Mitchell would greet every arriving plane to Molokai with an 'aloha' for every arriving passenger. He also helped us raise money on Molokai for the March of Dimes, the organization that sponsored our Birth Defects Center at Children's Hospital in Honolulu.

"In 1975, when our Healani women's crew decided we were going to do the first women's Molokai to Oahu crossing, I couldn't wait to tell Mitchell as I wanted his special greeting and blessings when we arrived. Well, not only was he there to greet us the day we arrived for the race, he had other locals there with flower leis and music. When he approached me he held a beautiful lei in one hand and a carved koa wood Palaoa in the other. I did not know at the time but since learned that historically the Palaoa is a curved whale tooth pendant that looks like a thick tongue curled up. It was typically carved of whalebone and sometimes human bone, and was adorned only by royalty. Its meaning is 'the exceptional warrior.' I remember Mitchell saying to me as he put the Palaoa around my neck, 'This will take you safely across to the finish.' And yes, indeed it did! We won that first race!

"In 2009, the Palaoa made its 30th crossing with me, tied onto the canoe underneath the canvas cover. It's displayed in my home in a special place along with many canoe racing medals. Every day I gaze at it and I'm so grateful for such an incredible gift and such wonderful memories."

It's clear that Doc Shay gives to others, to her community, and to society at large. Her humanness is very apparent. Shay is a bright, intelligent, and gifted woman. She is giving and concerned about others. She is competitive and has an enormous drive. Overcoming obstacles in which she had no control, like physical size and gender, are important contributors to her motivation and success. Realistic goal setting, training, enjoying physical activity, finding her passion, and loving life are some of her many assets. It's no wonder that this now 75-year-old female continues to achieve monumental accomplishments.

XVI

Goal Setting for 2010

With 50K and 50-mile events completed in 2009, I was now ready to set personal goals for 2010. My immediate 2010 running goals included the Jed Smith 50K in February, the Way Too Cool 50K in March, and the American River 50-mile run in April.

On a rainy sixth of February, I ventured to the Jed Smith 50K race to conquer my first goal for the year. Sue Smyth joined me at the race site and paced me for part of the run. On that particular run there were five 10K loops. Sue ran with me on the fourth loop and maybe the last mile or so of the fifth loop. I felt fairly strong during that last lap. I finished in 6 hours and 17 minutes.

On February 11, 2010, I finished a 15-mile, 3-hour training run on the trail. I performed my Bob Anderson stretching routine after my run and finished drinking the rest of my breakfast smoothie. The idea of a smoothie, which includes fresh fruits and vegetables along with a jalapeño chili and cayenne pepper, was introduced to me by my dear friend Jonathan Jordan. Soon after I finished my drink, I began thinking about doing the exact same run tomorrow but this time without my dog Digger, a two and a half year old white-haired Fox Terrier. During the run my shoulder was a little sore and I think it was related to Digger, since he's leashed during the run and tends to pull. The training run was a little different since I was concerned about my ability to increase my heart rate. I made sure that I did more uphill running.

On Thursday, the 17th of February, Linda and I left for San Diego to visit two of my dearest friends, one of whom was dying from cancer. Jonathan Jordan was diagnosed with cancer of the throat and neck in 2009. He completed chemo and radiation therapy in August of that same year. His goal was to run the Way Too Cool 50k on March 13, 2010. During his treatments he told me he wanted to envision a goal to help him through the therapies and deal better with his recovery. So we talked about the Way Too Cool Race and the training necessary for him to finish. We both knew that because of his health situation, he could use much more training time to build up his cardio and endurance. Saturday was going to be a good training day for him. Jonathan was both a great friend and a Ride & Tie partner. I still remember fondly our August 2008 completion and winning of the 100-mile Ride & Tie at Swanton in the Santa Cruz Mountains of California. Jonathan figured out the training trail run for that Saturday. We were joined by Jonathan's wife Tara, and Vince, a Ride & Tie friend whom I hadn't seen in years. Jonathan was 55 years of age, Tara 39, and Vince was in his 50s. Our three-hour plus run at Horse Thief Canyon was at the site of a previous Ride & Tie event with plenty of elevation change, making it great aerobic training. Jonathan ran extremely well and set the pace for the first loop and for most of the second loop. I was impressed with his speed and endurance. The last segment of our second loop was a steady, elevated climb. Tara and Vince ran faster while I stayed with Jonathan. After that run, it occurred to me that I needed to incorporate more hill work into my training. Several competitions loomed on the horizon: After competing in the 50k on March 13th, I planned to run the American River 50-mile on April 10th.

Linda and I had dinner with the Jordan's that evening. Sunday morning we left for our return home and on the way stopped and spent time with Denny and his wife Maria, which turned out to be the last time I would ever visit him.

I met Denny in the late 60s while teaching at Oakland community college. He was a psychologist who taught in the classroom next to mine. We developed a friendship that lasted over 40 years. We attended graduate school at Wayne State University. He was my friend and mentor. I looked up to him and admired his intelligence, brilliance and rebelliousness. He was also my teacher, role model, and confidant. I trusted him with my life. I loved him and miss being able to call him.

He had that special laugh that I will never forget. That man can never be replaced.

It was difficult and sad seeing my lifelong friend in a prolonged state of dying from pelvic cancer, yet I'm glad I got to see him if even for a short while. He had literally given up on life, and seemed to be waiting for the end. I didn't expect to ever see Denny alive again. His prognosis was not good. Sadness overwhelmed me as we said our goodbyes.

Linda and I arrived home late Sunday on Valentine's Day. On the 15th I ran a trail run of about 15 miles in a little over three hours. On the 16th I ran a loop that was about 15 miles. I was tired after the 15-mile trail run on Wednesday. Thinking about Thursday's trail run of 15 miles made me even more concerned about how tired I felt. Then I realized that I was still recovering from the Jed Smith 50K run I had completed on the 6th. Thursday morning I felt more rested and ready to go, and made a smoothie of two bananas, two apples, two oranges, and some yogurt. This mixture was basically for Linda. Then to the fruit base I added a jalapeño chili, cayenne pepper, carrot, broccoli, light salt, and ice. Linda didn't want any part of this combination. I might add that Jonathan suggested adding the peppers to my drink, which would assist with prostate issues. I ran this by my doctor but he was not convinced. To make sure I had enough energy, I took two capsules of Astaxanthin and ate a dish of oatmeal. Now all I had to do is my stretching routine and I would be ready for the run.

I had hoped my daughter Lori would join us but she unfortunately had a previous engagement. Lori and I had reconciliation during 2009. We took the opportunity to talk about the issues that were bothering her. She had a lot to say, and I mostly listened to the struggles she was experiencing with me. I attempted to be supportive; I listened and empathized with what she was going through. I had been hurt in years past and realized it would take some time for me to let down my guard, be there for her, and not be defensive.

My sister Beverly was the go-between for Lori and I during our difficult years. She worked very hard at helping me mend my relationship with my daughter and encouraged me over the years to reach out to Lori. Beverly came to California for a visit in the spring or summer each year. She split her time between and Lori and I. Beverly has been very helpful with repairing that relationship. Thank goodness I have a sister like her.

That spring, Beverly, Lori, my two grandsons Nick, Alex, and I traveled to Sunnyvale in Silicon Valley to meet my second cousins on my father's side of the family. I had not seen Diane, Linda or her husband Jeremy in quite some time and in fact, not since Linda and Jeremy's wedding. Lori made the contact and arranged for our visit. My cousins' father and mother, my first cousins Sherman and Lorraine, are family members who I love dearly. I still miss both of them. Sherman is 10 years older than me, which earns him the title of "big brother." I smile when I think about him and the things we did together.

One memory stands out, Sherman and Lorraine got married in Chicago, Illinois, when I was about 10 or 11 years old. My father and I attended the wedding by driving the 1950 Plymouth family car to the ceremony. On the return trip to Detroit, my father allowed me to drive. I remember sitting in the driver's seat while many of the people in the cars that passed us looked over to see if somebody was actually behind the wheel. I was not very tall at that age.

On the drive to Sunnyvale, I told Lori I wanted her in my life. I followed through by inviting her to parties and other social functions. So in 2010, I informed her about my running goals and asked her to attend these events. She said, "I'll put them on my calendar." Needless to say, our family trip and visit turned out to be terrific. I liked seeing my cousins and watching the interactions that took place between the adults.

Beverly left after her week-long visit and returned to Connecticut. I resumed my trail running in preparation for the Way Too Cool 50K in March. Jonathan Jordan was ambivalent about competing and I understood why. He loved to compete but his cancer limited his conditioning. I talked with his wife Tara and she believed it was a good idea for Jonathan to visit and participate in the run. She realized that he enjoyed his visits and mentally needed to do this for himself. Jonathan made a decision to run, and arrived the day before the event. I picked him up at the Sacramento Airport.

Somehow or other, Lori had something else scheduled on the morning of the Way Too Cool event. I asked Tony Brickel and Sue Smyth to pace me. Jonathan had Victoria Ordway for his pacer. As it turned out, Victoria met Jonathan at about the 6-mile marker at the Highway 49 crossing. He was ahead of me at that point. Jonathan and Victoria stayed in front of me all the way to the recycling center aid station some 15 to 16 miles into the run. That was typical of Jonathan, since he likes to beat me and win. I arrived at the aid station while Jonathan and Victoria were lingering about. I wasn't sure what they were doing, but I didn't believe their dawdling was related to me. That was my rationale for not stopping, and now I was in the lead. As I left the aid station, I yelled out, "You can catch up!"

Victoria had all kinds of energy and liked to run ahead, wait, run ahead, and then wait. They eventually caught up to me. After a mile or so, we all reached the turn-off called the Dead Truck trail (a defunct truck was abandoned near the trail). After running some 19 miles or so, Jonathan appeared tired and started to lag behind me.

When we reached Canyon Creek, I crossed the deep flowing creek with Jonathan close behind. Luckily some other young runners assisted me in traversing the raging creek, which was fast-running, thigh deep, and scary. Thank goodness for camaraderie within the running community. After climbing out of the creek, I headed toward the infamous Maine Bar climb a half-mile ahead. Jonathan hated this part of the run. I reached the top in front of him after a long, arduous and difficult climb. Tony met me near the top.

After passing the aid station, I saw Sue. I don't know how far Jonathan was behind because he was nowhere in sight. I thought silly me, Jonathan might be too tired to finish and therefore I didn't wait for him. Tony and I left, and as we started back on the trail, I looked back again and saw that Jonathan had made it to the aid station. I yelled,

"How are you doing?" He responded with, "I'm okay." So far so good. Jonathan continued to compete after running 20 some miles of difficult terrain. He was one tough dude. Once again, I was impressed with him.

Sue Smyth seemed to have good energy and was in front of Tony and me. We were proceeding down the Robie Trail on our way to the next aid station, which was now about 25 to 26 miles into the run. That next aid station was called Goat Hill, an appropriate name if you are a goat. When I reached the top of Goat Hill, Linda was there so I got my food supplies, filled my water bottles, and again headed back out on the trail. I looked around and saw Jonathan and Victoria. I yelled, "You're doing great!"

Tony and I continued down the trail. I didn't see Jonathan again until after I'd finished. He finished roughly nine to ten minutes behind Tony and me. After the run he confided that I helped him succeed. In truth, he would like to have beaten me. I was the motivation that helped him to plug away at the goal of finishing. He cannot, and would not, quit. Quitting is neither in his DNA nor in his psychological profile.

Another training run completed. I was not hurting and felt pretty good. I hoped that things would continue to go well for me; however, what is clear about life is that conditions always change.

What a surprise my third goal for 2010, the American River 50, turned out to be. It was now April and I was set. I was conditioned, at least I thought so, and would find out soon enough. This race began at Sacramento State University and finished in Auburn. The first 20 miles were uphill and adjacent to the cement bike trail that runs along the American River. The last 31 miles were difficult because the trail was dirt, rocky and steep. Steve Anderson planned to run with me the last 20 to 25 miles. Tony Brickel intended to run with me from Rattlesnake Bar to the finish line in Auburn, the last 10 miles or so. Lori and the boys were going to pick up Tony and drive him to Rattlesnake Bar. That was the pacing plan. Debbie Brickel was going to the finish line to meet all of us.

On race morning, Linda, Steve and I started out just fine but quickly returned home to change vehicles because the check engine light appeared in the van. We changed vehicles and luckily that didn't take too long. Linda, Steve, and I finally arrived late at the Sacramento State starting point. I got in line at the porta-potty and then noticed the race had already begun. There were no crowds at the race start because the runners were gone! So, I started out in last place. I didn't want to begin with too-fast a pace, and take the chance of burning out, so I did my best to stay evenly focused.

Linda and Steve were at some of the aid stations and they were a welcome sight. Steve met me at Beals Point on Folsom Lake (a short distance from Folsom Prison) and I was still doing okay. I was tired, but that's typical for these events. You're supposed to get tired. The temperature was cool, so I didn't want to be too cold nor too hot. I remembered the fable "Goldilocks and the Three Bears." Goldilocks would taste the porridge, try the beds, etc. and would pick the one that was just right. Me too; I had to get it right (like wearing the right gear). If not, I would pay for it one way or the other.

I eventually got to Rattlesnake Bar with Steve's help. He was great because he ran ahead, filled my water bottles, and got the food (power bars, GU, cooked potatoes, hot soup, pretzels and other available carbohydrates) that I needed to continue. This process worked perfectly for me.

Tony, Lori, Alex, Nick, and Linda were at Rattlesnake Bar. I yelled out, "Who's coming with me to the finish?" I was directing this message to my grandsons. Neither Alex nor Nick jumped up to volunteer. I purposely spent a little more time there than usual hoping that Alex would join in on the fun. Then all of a sudden Alex said, "I'll go with you, Grandpa." Lori looked surprised, although in retrospect she might have been terrified.

I said to Alex, "We have over nine miles to go and once we start, there is no turning back. The last three miles are straight up, it's called Cardiac Hill. You have to go the entire distance to the finish. No one can pick you up in between."

Alex was still firm in his conviction. He was dressed in a short sleeve T-shirt, pants, and non-running shoes. I said, "Okay, grab some water bottles because you have to drink. You might even want some Gatorade." He said emphatically, "No Gatorade." I might add that he wasn't wearing a belt, which meant that he was going to run with one hand holding onto his pants.

So off we went, the four of us—Tony, Steve, 15-year-old Alex, and me. Alex has a great personality and fits in extremely well with adults. He is outgoing, and carries on conversations with anyone near; what a charmer. He was often in the lead with a water bottle in one hand and the other keeping his pants up. We reached the next aid station and I told him, "Stock up on the food because you want to eat and make sure you drink." What teenager doesn't like to hear "eat all you want"? He got great praise and support from those at the aid station and the people we passed during the run. Then we reached the next aid station at Cardiac Hill, the name of which is certainly appropriate.

Steve was trashed at that point, but his only choice was to continue. I was feeling okay, Tony was feeling okay, and Alex was doing terrifically. We passed more runners and everybody said to Alex, "good job." Runners are familiar with the "good job" exchange between them. With about a mile and a half to go, I asked Tony to call Linda at the finish line and tell her to make sure the announcer acknowledged Alex over the loudspeaker. All I told Alex when we were close to the finish was that I would hold his hand as we crossed the line. Sure enough, the announcer acknowledged 15-year-old Alex and made a funny comment about me as we crossed the line.

This was a great experience for me to be able to run with my grandson. I was thrilled to death and thought it was one of those moments in time that I will always hold close to my heart. Alex did a great job, got a lot of good feedback, and I think he enjoyed himself. I took pride in being able to participate with him in an event that I love. I was pleased that my daughter was present and allowed Alex to participate with me. Things were going well in 2010. And it was still only April.

And now, some words from Alex. "Pacing for my Grandpa was a really cool experience because I got to see him in his natural element. When you are just there supporting him on the sidelines, you don't get a real idea of the skill and effort it takes to participate in this kind of sport. I am proud of my Grandpa for running in these events, because they are strenuous, even for younger people like me, and to see him doing it is great. I am glad that he has introduced me into the world of running, because it's a great sport. As a suburban kid, I'm not that familiar with the natural beauty of the great outdoors and because of my somewhat limited attention span, pacing my Grandpa was a perfect mixture of sightseeing and exercise. I got to spend some quality time with my Grandpa doing something he loves. The fun of running seems to slowly be creeping up on me, as well as getting some views of the great outdoors. I was filled with pride as my Grandpa crossed the finish line, because although it was just another race to him, spending those final 10 miles with him bonded us much better as grandfather and grandson.

One of my tasks was to develop a different relationship with my grandsons. I only knew one grandfather growing up, since the other one died when I was very young. My mother's father, my grandma, and my aunt lived close by. What I remember most are a few conversations I had with my maternal grandpa. He was a good-looking man and lived until the age of 93. One of the things he told me was that our economic system is upside down. In his opinion, the younger folks should have more sums of money because that's when they needed it most. He believed that when he got older he required less money to get by. He also had a good firm handshake. That grip demonstrated his strength and it was important for him to show it.

On August 5th, a Thursday, I received a call from Jennifer Tiscornia, Jim Steere's youngest daughter. She simply said, "Jim passed Tuesday evening." I didn't believe her at first. Jennifer said, "D'Ann wanted you to know because Jim referred to you as his buddy." We talked some more and she told me there was going to be a memorial in Petaluma.

What a shock! I didn't want to believe that he had died. Just that June, Jim (at age 85) had teamed up with his son Thom at the 40th Ride & Tie championship—and they finished. I had just talked to Jim the Thursday prior on July 29.

On that Thursday evening, Jim and I talked about a presentation he was going to make on behalf of his mother's sculptural art that she had crafted over the years. He claimed he was having difficulty in writing his presentation. I told him, "You have a wealth of information, Jim." He said, "I know, I'm still having trouble, but I'll get it done." I thought he sounded a little tired, but it was late and I didn't think much more about it. What is clear is that Jim lived a full life right up until the end. He continued to compete. What a testimony to a wonderful, intelligent, passionate, and giving human being.

Jim was to be our head vet for the run and Ride & Tie in Cool, September 17th and 18th. Instead, we honored James Henry Steere in a number of ways, including adding "Jim Steere's extended family" to the front of our T-shirts. We also created a memorial trophy in honor of Dr. Steere. This trophy includes the winning team for the last five years on our long course and is displayed by our local sponsors. We invited Jim's wife D'Ann and the Steere family to the Ride & Tie.

At the event, Thom Steere and wife Becky competed in the 17-mile event along with Robert and Leslie Steere. Jim's youngest daughter Jennifer brought the horses. D'Ann attended and was gracious. Friday night at the potluck we honored Jim and his family with a number of testimonials. I was emotional when I gave mine, and certainly the family was also emotional. I was happy to be able to give something back to them in honor of their father and husband as Jim gave so much to me. He was quite the man, and I considered him to be a wise sage, I miss him dearly.

XVII

Ms. Independent, Sammie Stanbro:
Paddler of the World

While interviewing athletes for my book, I asked Doc Shay to refer me to people who knew about her accomplishments. One of the names she gave me was Sammie Stanbro. As it turned out, Sammie not only provided great input about Doc Shay, she also had an intriguing story of her own. I refer to her as Ms. Independent.

Sammie Stanbro is about 5 feet 9-1/2 inches tall and weighs approximately 145 pounds. She was born on March 5, 1945, in Oakland, California. Her mother Joanne married Robert, and he journeyed to the Pacific to serve in the U.S. Marines during World War II. Joanne and her child didn't live in Oakland very long before moving to San Diego.

In San Diego, Sammie became independent as a result of consistently being left alone; her mother worked to support them. Sammie recalled fondly that in elementary school years, she rode her bike, surfed and swam a lot. She loved horses and was referred to as "horse face" by her friends. Some friends! She was absolutely horse crazy, and fortunately for her there was a stable nearby. She would ride her bicycle to the stable, clean stalls, and ride horses as a reward for her labor. Sammie honed her equestrian skills and was trained in both English and Western styles of riding. She competed in gymkhana, fast-paced games like barrel racing and pole bending, as well as in jumping events. Even at this point in her life she was competitive, competent, and extremely active. And along the way she learned self-reliance.

Although she was an average student in elementary school, Sammie was exceptional at art, specifically drawing and painting. She received numerous compliments about her creativity, and according to her, "It got me through school." It wasn't until she was 16 years old that she met her father for the first time; her parents divorced when Robert returned home after the war ended.

Later on, Sammie learned more about her father's deeds as a Marine during the war. Her father, while on the island of Iwo Jima, received a telegraph that simply stated, "You have a daughter." Robert was wounded in action, but he was the lucky one, many of his battalion buddies died during battle. In talking about her father, Sammie mentioned the book, "Flags of Our Fathers," and recalled that these men didn't talk about the horrors of war. She never had a conversation about the World War II conflict with her father, but he did show her a map and a Japanese flag. She also remembered seeing a picture of Iwo Jima on his bedroom wall. She added, "If only I could talk to him about the war." To this day Sammie regrets not having that conversation with her dad. She definitely regrets not being close to her father.

Sammie talked about spending time with her grandparents. She claimed that her grandfather was her male figure and that she admired them both. Her grandfather built Methodist churches and moved around a lot, especially throughout Northern California. Her mother remarried after Sammie left home. She recalled that her mother was an attractive, independent and wonderful woman. Sammie reported that, "She taught me that I can do anything I want to." Her mother had boyfriends who were scuba divers and who piloted planes. So Sammie also enjoyed the adventures of scuba and flying to various water locations.

It's important to note that a medical condition concerning Sammie's knees had a dramatic affect on Sammie's personality. As a young teenager, her kneecaps slid back and forth, and a doctor declared that kneecap surgery was necessary. No one in that era ever argued with medical opinion. As a result she had "successful surgery," only to discover that she was not able to run, skip, or jump. Today, removing one's kneecaps is never done. Thank goodness for that.

Regardless, Sammie adapted and worked on making her upper body strong. The theme of self-reliance and overcoming obstacles was strongly ingrained in her, in part thanks to the knee surgery and Sammie's upbringing. She disliked having to ask anyone for assistance and took pride in doing things herself like running her six acre coffee farm. At one point she even fixed the plumbing in her bathroom by herself.

Sammie wanted to see the Barrier Reef in Australia so her first goal was to get to Hawaii. After completing two years of college, she purchased a boat ticket and ventured off to Hawaii. At that time, Don Ho was just getting started with his singing career. Sammie remembered spending a lot of time at Duke Kahanamoku's in Honolulu where Don Ho was performing, since her new friends were dating members of the band.

While hanging out in Hawaii, Sammie met a yacht owner who was going to Australia to race in the famous Sydney-to-Hobart event. This event was one of the largest yacht races in the world, and the boats raced in treacherous waters. During that time, women generally were not allowed to be part of the crew. However, yacht owner Thompson said, "You make it to Australia, and I'll take you on as crew."

For the next year Sammie worked and saved her money to make the trip to Australia. She eventually reached the "Land Down Under" after first spending time in Japan and Hong Kong. She added that traveling by boat back then was not only inexpensive, but was also a wonderful introduction to that mode of travel.

After arriving in Australia, she found out that Thompson's yacht was actually in New Zealand. She boarded another ship and for a $50 ticket reached New Zealand. After searching for the yacht owner, she found him and shouted out, "Hey, do I still have a job?" It turned out the yacht was without a mast and the owner's crew was short. What a lucky moment, and for the next two and a half years Sammie sailed the Pacific, chalking up many wonderful adventures.

An example of Sammie's independent, self-reliant, and adventurous spirit was portrayed at 21 years of age in 1966. That year she was one of three women in the Sydney-Hobart yacht race which hosted 60-plus yachts. During that race, she was caught in a deadly storm in which several crew members were killed. There was a combination of 90 mph winds and 60 feet of towering seas which flipped seasoned racing yachts, broke their masts and swamped the boats. The following narrative is taken from her 'ship's log' of a terrible and terrifying experience while on the Nam Sang, the racing yacht that was her home and transportation for two years in the South Pacific and Tasman Ocean rim waters.

Sammie's log read: "80 mile-per-hour gusts, three days out of Sydney, Australia. The gale of this Tasmanian hurricane was so wild it would toss the beautiful solid gold platter around like a cork. We reefed the Nam and dropped the sea anchor. All the vents were stuffed with towels, everything was lashed down and water was everywhere. I was below deck, cold and miserable. Bilges were pumped regularly; the three sick crew members were cared for in the cold deck below. The only way to get warm was by lying next to another crew member.

"The boat was being swamped as a huge wave came from the stern and tore heavy railings and the solid teak masts. The magnificent ship's wheel was dashed to bits and the large stainless steel compass binnacle was severed. Life rafts were at the ready in the main salon and all life jackets ready to slip on at any moment. The six crew people who were handling the boat were below wondering, "what next?" Then there was silence, scary-still, quiet gray sky and sea. The feeling was eerie but it felt good when the bashing stopped. It didn't last long, only a couple of minutes, and then it all started in again. Out came the emergency tiller, and one-half-hour watches took all our energy. We went back to Australia for repairs and a new stainless wheel. Eight days at sea in a trusted yacht with six able crew members."

This crew realized they just had to keep going no matter what happened next. This was an extraordinary experience for this young woman, and turned out to be the ultimate teacher for her to "never give up." Sammy added that she logged about 12,000 miles in the Pacific and Tasman before turning age 23.

In 1969, Sammie was in a relationship with her Australian boyfriend when her friends suggested that she should meet this man, a navigator, from San Diego. As it turned out, she did indeed meet Phil the navigator, who was planning a trip to Japan. He was going to visit the island, purchase a motorcycle, and explore the land and culture for a few months. Phil invited Sammie to join him on this adventure. Her boyfriend at the time said, "You always follow the sun."

So Sammie was off to Japan in a heartbeat. This adventure turned romantic and she married Phil at the end of 1969 in San Diego with both families in attendance.

In 1973, Sammie, Phil, and baby Joshua moved to Northern California where they purchased 85 acres of land and built their house. Sammie had fruit orchards, horses, fir, pine, and oak trees with a river running through the property. Sammie raised chickens for food, she even had a Nubian goat for yogurt, cheese, and of course milk. She was becoming independent, self taught, and an expert at butchering. While on the ranch, Sammie was a substitute teacher and Phil was a school administrator. In 1983, Phil had a midlife crisis, made a career change, and relocated the family to Oregon where second son Orion was born. While in Oregon, they procured an old house on Lake Oswego, purchased a sailboat, and Sammie was back on the water, this time paddling.

The Stanbro family moved to Hawaii in the late 1990s. Phil was diagnosed with prostate cancer and died in 2001. Shortly after his death, Sammie found herself off the Kona shores of the Big Island of Hawaii, paddling in her son's one man canoe. She was going out to sea, and coming towards the shore were a crew team of senior women in an outrigger canoe. She called out to them, "That looks like fun!" Their reply was, "It is! Why don't you come out with us?" Before Sammie could reply, one crew member shouted out, "How old are you?" Sammie yelled back, "I just turned 55." That was absolutely what these mature women wanted to hear.

Thus began a new life for Sammie; new sport, new group of friends, and a new direction in life. "It gets me up in the morning and fills a huge void in my life," reflected Sammie. "My husband and I were soul mates and at that time I didn't have a big support system. It gave me direction and filled the requirement of my time. I had to be there for training."

Being in crisis, experiencing grief and loss, being vulnerable, setting the stage for a new beginning and new lifestyle, Sammie was going through all this. But her sense of adventure, competitive nature, athletic ability, love of the water, and her mental and physical prowess all helped Sammie find a new, challenging, and enriching way to live. Once again we recognize how a personal life crisis results in an emotional disequilibrium, and can allow certain individuals to eventually rebalance and experience a positive and fulfilling growth.

Sammie has developed strong upper body strength, and she relies on that strength in competition, especially when another boat is in front of her. When another outrigger is in front of her in a competition, the spirited nature of this woman rises to the surface and she begins to push her physical limits. For Sammie, this is the moment the race begins.

In 2008 and 2009 Sammie raced from Molokai to Oahu as part of the Pure Light Racing Team in the men's Molokai race event. This adaptive team consisted of the blind, paraplegics, and amputees, who with courage and self determination are inspiring to see. In addition, Sammie has completed nine women's Molokai to Oahu Outrigger Canoe races.

In 2009, she raced in the Cook Islands Outrigger Canoe races. When she heard that a Tahitian team was looking for a male paddler 50 years of age or older, Sammie said, "I'm interested, but I'm not a male!" After the Tahitian teammates learned that her qualifications included completing two men's Molokai races, "They grabbed me up," Sammie smiled. "I tucked my long blonde hair under my hat so not to be noticed, what a disguise!"

She also paddled in the Regatta in the mixed men and women's team as well as women's events representing the Keauhou Canoe Club. She loves being able to participate and compete with all paddlers from the other islands. Today she has won 11 state championships. However, it takes a team to win and the senior members of the Keahou Canoe Club are unequaled. "Competitor" just might be her middle name. Older, or should I say, young-at-heart athletes have this competitor spirit stamped in their character.

Sammie looks youthful, and her esprit is certainly that of a young person. She feels pride and satisfaction when people are surprised to discover her 'youthful' age.

Sammie shared more of her thoughts on paddling . . . "The exhilaration of moving as one with a wave is thrilling; the powerful stroke of nature is all-consuming. My hand ripping through the ocean each time I stroke, the grab of the blade, the challenge of learning how to be the most efficient with my body, technique, strength, and mental focus, all blend to make me one with the canoe.

"The Outrigger canoe is a design that has evolved over the centuries to be efficient and more recently, fast. A traditional Koa Outrigger gives such pleasure to the eye, a work of art instilled with Manna (power) . . . when she moves she feels alive.

"Working together as a team, six crew members ideally move as one even though each has a different job. Timing is exact, the canoe lifts and glides with the thrust of power; the feeling is pure pleasure.

"For our Pure Light adaptive crew the experience is heightened because we get the feel of motion and speed that we can no longer get with the use of our legs. Our big open ocean races are dangerous, we rely on crew members to be there for each other; similar to my sailing days, we become sisters and brothers rising to the challenge of the sea.

"The canoe will teach you about yourself and offer you the opportunity for growth mentally as well as physically . . . and it is so much fun!"

Her paddler teammates and friends all have college degrees and are professional women. Sammie is not a recreational paddler, but she is certainly a serious athlete. She has won many medals, competed in a number of state championships, and is a member of the Hawaiian Canoe Racing Association.

Sammie received paddling instructions from a top paddler, who taught her the Tahitian stroke. This specific stroke helped her become more efficient so she could "paddle all day." Sammie told me that when you are paddling efficiently, you can feel it, the connection between the ocean and outrigger canoe. This sounds similar to 'being in the zone' or 'being one with your horse' that other athletes talk about.

When one is paddling in competition, there is no idle talk. Sammie believes that women paddlers have humility, which is important to being a good sport. Being gracious and congratulating other paddlers is the proper etiquette in this sport. "You don't rub it in" when you win, according to Sammie. During her Cook Island paddling adventure, she received a great compliment from 40 year old Lisa Curry, three-time Olympic swimmer from Australia. Lisa said, "I would do anything to be able to do what you do at your age, you're my idol" The ultimate compliment!

Currently, Sammie resides in Kona on the big island. She and Phil designed and built an unusual three-story island home. Many of its recycled components came from all over the world. The home is situated in the middle of six acres surrounded by avocado and coffee trees. In fact, her home is used as a tourist destination. Outstanding Island chefs create Hawaiian dinner delights for people on tour at Sammie's home.

When not on the water paddling, Sammie is taking care of her coffee trees. The most challenging part of being a coffee plantation owner is the harvest. From October through January you'll find her picking coffee beans, putting them in 50-pound bags and taking them to market.

It's clear that Sammie transformed her physical handicap with her knees into a physical advantage. She is strong physically, and in her own words "can paddle all day." Her mental toughness is also apparent as she strives to be the best. She's a fierce competitor, sets and accomplishes goals, and is one motivated lady. She is involved in local island politics and gives back to the community. Her sons and grandchildren are her delights and Sammie has been an excellent role model. She's developed an extended family in the world of paddling, and continues to seek adventure and new challenges. Sammie is one terrific paddler, and one beautiful human being.

XVIII

The Ultimate Caretaker:
Beverlee Bentley, Gold Medal Rower

Young Beverlee Bentley is another remarkable female athlete. She is a 72-year-old married woman who lives in Mill Valley, California. She is 5-feet 9-inches tall and weighs approximately 140 pounds, and was born in the small mining town of Cobalt, Ontario, Canada on August 2, 1938. For the last 10 years, she has competed in rowing regatta national and local competitions. The Beverlee of today is different from the Beverlee of the past. This is her story and the remarkable changes she's encountered over the years. Her philosophy is, "If the door opens, make sure you go through it."

On March 4, 1994 Beverlee's 57-year-old husband Bill was downhill skiing at Alpine Village, a ski resort in the Sierra Nevada Mountains. Bill was quite the athlete. In addition to being a Black Diamond skier, he rode mountain bikes, ran marathons, and was in good physical shape. Years prior to this benchmark day, he sustained a neck injury while body surfing at Stinson Beach in California's Marin County and recovered fully from that accident.

On that March day, the snow was soft and Bill was near the bottom of the ski slope after skiing down from Alpine's most difficult run. He was skiing with a friend and they were planning on another run. Bill turned his head to say something to his friend when his ski caught an edge. Bill fell and severed his spinal cord at C5 and C6. This horrifying and tragic accident dramatically changed the lives of Bill and Beverlee Bentley.

Bill is now totally dependent on his wife. Some of Beverlee's responsibilities include turning him over in bed while making sure the sheets are without wrinkles so he won't get bed sores. She washes his face and hands every day, as well as emptying and washing his catheter bag. She feeds him and provides range-of-motion stretching exercises daily. She works with his legs, ankles, arms, and fingers, making sure to rotate and bend his body parts. She gets him out of bed by pulling his legs over the side while she rolls him onto his side in order to prop him up in a sitting position. She uses a transfer belt to take him from the bed to his $25,000 electric wheelchair. She brushes his teeth and dresses him. His arms can move slightly but his fingers can't. She places rubber tips on his fingers so he is able to turn the pages of the newspaper. This is a brief glimpse into the daily life of the Bentleys.

Beverlee talked about how difficult that first year after the accident was for her. She had nightmares and cried herself to sleep because of the major changes in her life. Prior to this accident, Beverlee fantasized about the two of them traveling together, returning to college to study anthropology, and maybe even getting her degree during her retirement years.

She didn't want to look after Bill. Her life was turned upside down and her mental and emotional states were in disarray. After much turmoil and soul-searching, she reached a decision. "I couldn't leave him," she reports, "and I knew I had to deal with Bill in the here and now."

Later on Beverlee realized that she needed something more in her life than being a caretaker. A friend suggested that they attend a "learn to row" workshop. She accompanied her friend to that morning workshop, in part because the morning time was a good time for her to be away from Bill. Beverlee believes that rowing answered her many needs for a healthy life—exercise, camaraderie, meditation, and focus. She comments that, "I really love rowing. It keeps me strong and I am blessed I have sport and exercise in my life."

Beverlee's hometown is Toronto, Canada. She is the oldest child in her family and has a fraternal twin sister, Marie. She remembers that she competed with Marie in a "covert" way. Summers were spent at a nearby lake, and Beverlee made sure to beat Marie when the two of them swam together, although she didn't admit to actually racing her sister. She did say that Marie told her, "I'm smarter than you," and there is no doubt that competition existed between the girls.

During Beverlee's high school years, she was self-conscious and believed that she was too tall and ugly compared to her twin. She was struggling with her self-image and didn't feel as good or as pretty as the other girls. Beverlee attended a girl's Catholic high school and played on the basketball team. Her memory is dim about that time in her life. She didn't think basketball was a big deal, and commented, "The uniforms were ugly," but she played guard on the basketball team. In those days, girls' basketball was played differently than it is now and guards only used two thirds of the basketball court. She stayed after school, practiced, and played against other high school girls' teams. It's not a surprise that Beverlee downplayed her sports involvement. Her parents didn't attend any of her games or comment about her participation in basketball. She didn't get validation from her parents, so it was difficult to be proud of her accomplishments. She participated in intramural track and competed as a long jumper. She was a member of the choir and liked singing. She believed that if it were not for her friend Pat Palmer, she might not have played basketball. "Pat was athletic and liked sports," remembers Beverlee. "Sports were not encouraged by the nuns in parochial high school either."

Beverlee recently contacted Pat Palmer. I asked Beverlee to have Pat refresh her memory about her high school days. Pat reminded her about playing basketball and volleyball in high school. It was clear that Beverlee's family was not particularly interested in her sports prowess but it was a totally different story at Pat's house. Her parents were athletic and maintained a keen interest in Pat and her game dynamics.

Beverlee loves rowing, is knowledgeable about a lot of the different techniques, and likes to race. If there is a boat in front of her, "I want to catch up or be in front of the other rowers," says Beverlee, "even if the others are not racing. I race all the time. Winning is a priority for me."

Beverlee believes that she was her father's favorite among the four girls. She pleased him, was helpful, obedient, and gave him no grief. Beverlee's sister Marie said, "You are his favorite, and you're a goody two shoes." Marie, the rebel, wanted everyone to do things her way. There was one fight that Marie had with her father about going to a high school dance. Her father did not let Marie go to the dance at age 15. Beverlee told me, "I never wanted to go to a dance; I wasn't even interested in boys."

After completing high school, Beverlee attended St. Michael's nursing school. A couple of friends from nursing school left Canada to seek work in San Francisco, where, at the age of 21, Beverlee applied for a nursing job. At first, the visit was supposed to be for a few months so Beverlee could be with her friends. She joined three of her friends in a two-bedroom apartment that came with two double beds. "Back then we accepted that arrangement as being normal," states Beverlee. She stayed for three years and then returned home to care for her ill mother. Her mother had a heart attack and passed away in 1964. Beverlee knows about being a caregiver; she's had practice.

In 1964, Beverlee married Bill. She gave birth to Christian in 1965, Eric in 1968, Craig in 1969, Adam in 1971, and Jessica in 1974. She stopped working as a nurse about three months after Christian's birth. Having three young boys in diapers turned out to be a full-time job. She remembers how she spent her time: meals, cleaning, laundry, cooking, driving, and gardening. "I worked morning to night," reports Beverlee. "I was on a treadmill. I didn't reflect much about these years, even though I was pretty reactive at that time." She definitely wins the award as the traditional homemaker.

In the 1980s, life became more difficult for Beverlee and the family. Craig got into trouble with drugs, and Beverlee became aware of Bill's difficulties with alcohol. In 1986 things got even worse and Beverlee and Bill separated for about four months and then reconciled. During the separation, she became more assertive, employed less denial, and took more responsibility for her part in the co-dependency dynamics. She read self-help books, had psychotherapy interventions, took college classes, and started walking for about an hour a day.

Beverlee returned to nursing in 1990 and took a hospital position in orthopedics. Beverlee was in a midlife crisis and it wasn't until she turned about 50 that things began to change in a positive way for her. She started to find more of a sense of self and in return, her marriage was better. Prior to this time, she was the "super mom" and all things to all people. The only thing that was missing was her own sense of what she needed. She never reflected on what was important to her. Her direction and focus were on the family and everyone else. She was similar to her mother in many ways, but things began to slowly change. Her self-esteem improved, and she found a focus. Beverlee became more self-directed, and she was no longer selfless.

Beverlee expects to live somewhere between 90 and 100 years of age, and plans to be active until she dies. She believes that doing things for others enriches her life and increases her own self-worth, and she feels happy and satisfied with her current life. She also believes that staying in touch with friends, exercise, music and making plans are important components to aging gracefully. She keeps a positive outlook because a negative outlook, "robs you of many things, including energy." She would like to have engraved on her tombstone, "You'll have to mind your own business now—because I'm out of here."

Beverlee believes it's important to realize that it is never too late to start a sport, even if one's history suggests otherwise. She acknowledges that people are becoming more active as they age. For her, rowing was important in her life because she learned something new. She also learned that she can compete with others, and that winning is very inspiring for her. She is currently more upfront with the idea of wanting to triumph, and giving herself permission to win.

Beverlee receives overwhelming support for her rowing from friends and teammates, although she doesn't request that friends come to her races because rowing is not a great spectator sport. Husband Bill has become a cheerleader which helps reinforce her continuing to row. Her children also are supportive and always ask about her rowing activities.

At the Gold Rush Masters Regatta at Lake Natoma in Northern California on the 22nd of May, 2010, Beverlee competed in a mixed quad (two men and two women), a double, and a mixed double. She came in first in a single, first in the double and fourth in the mixed quad. These distances were 1000-meters and were called sprints. Beverlee was worried prior to these races, afraid that she might not be able to compete decently. She had a minor injury that affected her ability to train. As it turned out, while in Hawaii her mental training suffered too: "I never felt old before; is this how old people feel?" These worries vanished, for the time being, after she performed well at Lake Natoma. The psychological line between feeling young and vibrant versus feeling vulnerable and old is fragile. One does not always feel or think that one is invincible. The realities of aging are present and it is difficult to deny them all the time.

Later in the year, Beverlee thought about competing in the Southwest Regional's at Lake Merritt in Oakland, California, and in the fall at the World Games in Canada. Her dilemma about traveling to Canada was associated with the expense and whether to take Bill with her. If she didn't take Bill, then she was likely to worry about him. If she took him, then she would be more comfortable and likely spend more time visiting with friends, teammates, and family. Ultimately, Beverlee decided not to attend the event.

One story Beverlee likes to tell is about when she drove with Bill from Mill Valley, California, to Victoria, British Columbia, for a Canadian Masters national competition. They arrived a day early, and Beverlee took a walk on the boat dock where the launching for the races was to take place. She was getting a head start in preparing for the races. Beverlee was walking down the ramp, looking ahead, when she fell suddenly because she missed a step at the bottom. She just sat on the dock and prayed that she didn't break any bones, all the while hoping that she could even just get up and walk. After a few minutes of pain and contemplation, she knew she had sprained her ankle. She slowly got up on her feet, thankful she could walk at all. She had signed up for five races, and on top of that, was the only person who could transfer and care for Bill. Beverlee knew she had to be okay. She iced her ankle the entire day and even purchased a brace for it. She was in agony and worried about whether or not she should scratch from the competition.

The next day, she seemed better and was able to function. Then her singles race came up and so did the wind. She didn't scratch; she entered and captured a gold medal. Beverlee was overjoyed! She felt such relief and elation.

After five years of rowing, Beverlee became more serious about the sport. That's when the training became more demanding. She rowed on the water or indoors with a rowing machine six days a week for about an hour and a half each day. She also lifted weights and performed core strengthening exercises two to three times a week.

Currently, Beverlee rides a bike for cross-training as she is unable to run or hike because of an arthritic knee. She is not on any medication and isn't restricted in any other way. She feels physically and mentally great and still loves to compete. She believes that her exercises help her remain strong for Bill, who recently asked her, "How long do you think you can continue to hold me and help me like you do?"

Thank goodness Beverley found that rowing, exercise, goal setting, raising her level of aspiration, following through, and competition allow her to be more complete as a person. She is not just a homemaker or caregiver. She is much more, and a pleasure to be around. She continues to be in the process of her own evolution, realizing the importance of rowing in her development and self-fulfillment.

XIX

The Why Questions Are Answered

I have learned many insights along this journey, and as a psychologist and senior athlete who competes in ultra-sports, I was intrigued by other's motivations as well as my own.

I began this project in February 2009. I quickly became more cognizant of articles and information about aging individuals, older athletes, and the benefits of exercise. I read a book by Lee Berquist entitled, "Second Wind: The Rise of the Ageless Athlete." In his book, he depicts stories of older athletes. Before reading this book, I thought "he beat me to the punch." But after reading his book, I realized my focus was different from his, and would provide answers to questions regarding the underlying motivation of the older athlete in extreme and unusual sports. I wanted to better understand what drives this unique athlete.

In reading the Wall Street Journal, I noticed there is a section of the newspaper titled "Personal Journal" with articles pertaining to health and wellness. A few of the titles include: "Spinning Blood Isn't Just for Athletes," "New Exercise Goal: 60 Minutes a Day," "Tough New Workout Gear That Goes Easy on the Joints," and the "Winter Olympics." This paper also covers college and professional football, collegiate and professional basketball, baseball, national and international soccer and golf. There is also extensive coverage of the Winter Olympic Games.

Not to be outdone by the Wall Street Journal, the New York Times has articles such as "Seeing Old Age as a Never-Ending Adventure," "The Human Body Is Built for Distance," and "Does Exercise Really Keep Us Healthy?" Time Magazine, on its August 17, 2009 cover, had a photograph of a young woman on a treadmill eyeing a cupcake. Below the cupcake is the article title, "The Myth About Exercise" with the subhead, "Of course it's good for you, but it won't make you lose weight. Why it's what you eat that really counts."

The August 2009 Self magazine sported a photograph of an athletic-looking 41-year-old Dana Torres. The associated article is titled, "What's Age Got to Do with It?" According to Dana, age has nothing to do with it. She became the oldest swimmer ever (at age 41) to win a Gold Medal at the Summer Olympic Games. In her article, she gives seven tips to uncover the strongest and sexiest self ever.

A 2010 issue of Time Magazine lists the 100 most influential people in the world and features older individuals like President Bill Clinton; Lee Kuan Yew, the prime minister of Singapore; and Edna Foa, a psychologist who developed a therapeutic approach to treat PTSD (post traumatic stress disorder). In its July 19, 2010 issue this magazine featured Robert Butler, founder of the International Longevity Center. His organization is dedicated to promoting healthy aging. He campaigned against ageism and dealt with the misconceptions and ignorance that fuel age prejudice. He believes that the elderly can be as productive, engaged, open to new ideas, and fun as younger people. By no means is my list exhaustive.

PBS television broadcasts a program called Health Quest. This program features presentations such as healthy eating, seniors employing cognitive exercises and its relation to Alzheimer's, and meditation for healthy living. Health and exercise are both covered by written and visual media. As you can see, topics of health and exercise are extremely popular today.

I am not a typical 71-year-old. My definition of exercise is different from most individuals, especially within my age group. Periodically, I sustain an injury from over use and seek assistance from Jim Kreutz, a local physical therapist. At his rehabilitation center, I typically meet many senior men and women. I can clearly tell that my workouts and rehabilitation regime are very different from my peers. My rehabilitation and exercise program is much more strenuous. I sweat a lot and I like it.

The result of my physical activities is that I have had the pleasure and fortune of meeting exceptional, positive thinking, inspirational, and wonderful human beings. Getting to know these men and women has greatly enriched my life. I am proud and flattered to have become friends with the people you have read about in these pages. There is pain too; the loss of Jim Steere hurts. A loss like that is never replaced. He became a good friend and I miss him greatly. I can't say enough about that man.

From my perspective and understanding, it is clear that genetics play only a part in the story of aging for these athletes. For some, parents provided a great model for physical activity, sports, and self-reliance. Doc Shay, Sammie, and Jim Steere quickly come to mind. Their parents were athletic, active, and provided positive feedback to their children. They walked the walk and encouraged their children to do so as well. These parents provided a framework, an expertise, for their children's behavior and illustrated a healthy way to live one's life.

I completely understand that parents are not the only role models in one's life. Professional athletes like Doak Walker, the Detroit Lions halfback in the 1950s, come to mind. He is my favorite football player and I enjoyed listening to the Detroit Lions football games announced by Van Patrick on the radio every Sunday during the season. Mr. Walker is a person who I admired, looked up to, and wanted to emulate. He is my hero. Other outstanding runners and an older brother were significant models for Russ Kiernan and played a part in his success. We identify with our role models and they are extremely important to us.

One's environment seems to play a major role in what we become, and contributes to our unique style of life. It's no surprise that Doc Shay, who grew up near the Gulf of Mexico, moved to Hawaii and still lives on the Big Island there. Playing near and on the water for Doc Shay is as natural as Jim Steere riding horses all over the desert, mountains and hills of California. Beverlee Bentley lived near the water in the province of Ontario and then moved to the lovely San Francisco Bay Area. It's no surprise that she's a rower in Marin County. What about Jack Sholl growing up near the Schuylkill River in Philadelphia, dropping out of high school to work in the shipyards, and meeting his future wife while rowing? It is easy to understand why he is still involved in a water sport.

Playing sports, liking physical activity, and having fun are important components in our lives. Doc Shay, Sammie, Beverlee, Lew, Russ, Jim, and I loved playing outdoors.

We played as kids and still play outdoors even today. Fun, enjoyment, play, and sports go together. We like sports for reasons that pertain to our ego, our 'self.' If sports were not rewarding and we didn't enjoy the activity, we might discontinue this lifestyle. It is important to play, enjoy, and have fun. Remember, it's all about the game. We certainly don't do it for the money.

Competitiveness has played an important part in man's development and in his history. We are hardwired for survival which means we have had to compete. In fact, society gives us awards like money, fame, or a medal for beating our rivals. Receiving an award from another is called extrinsic reinforcement. On the other hand, when we accomplish something like an activity that is pleasing or satisfying in and of itself, we call that intrinsic reinforcement. Obviously, in competition both intrinsic and extrinsic rewards occur.

Each one of us is highly competitive. Does play influence competitiveness, or does competitiveness influence play? One can make an argument that early childhood parental experiences play a significant part in the development of competitiveness. That part is clear. What is also apparent is that the involvement in sports gives the individual an opportunity to express that healthy competitiveness.

All of us who compete are motivated and supported by the extended family and community that evolve from these sports. The need for affiliation is designated as secondary and not as strong as the primary drive for food. However, studies have shown that being a part of a group and having a human connection are major, important, mental health components. We live longer, are healthier, happier, and more content when that human need is met.

Erik Erikson, a famous psychoanalyst wrote about "generativity," defined as giving to, taking care of, and guiding others. He theorizes it is one of the major stages in man's development. Looking at the lives of these athletic people, it is apparent that they give back to society. One of Doc Shay's favorite movies, "Pay It Forward," has now become her personal motto. She donates time, expertise, and gives medical supplies to those less fortunate. Russ Kiernan coaches track and is an elementary school teacher. Jim Steere was significantly involved in the Marin Hospice in his later years. Lew Hollander wrote a novella about climate change and recommendations to deal with this problem and Beverlee Bentley chooses to be a full time caretaker.

Giving to others, helping others, and extending oneself are character traits of these human athletes. In other words, social interest and being a contributing member of the community are important and necessary for these types of athletes. Humanness is an important and necessary component in the development of the family of man.

Overcoming loss or divorce and still moving forward in a positive and healthy way characterize many of these athletes. Did divorce interfere in a negative way with Doc Shay, Jim Steere, Lew, or me? No! In fact, it seems that the emotional trauma of divorce didn't impair any of us in the long term. It obviously didn't cripple us nor did it stigmatize us in our 'journey with self.' It seems that we got stronger and developmentally became healthier. In other words, getting rid of the negative irritant or non-working relationship proved beneficial. I'm suggesting that extricating or minimizing stress in one's life is important and necessary for growth, health, and well-being.

Likewise, losing loved ones, like Sammie and Russ did, provided them with an opportunity for new experiences and facilitated their personal journey and development. These two individuals overcame the trauma associated with the loss of a significant other. Fortunately for them, it did not get in their way of living their lives in a more fulfilling manner. Their grit, strength, perseverance, and drive are apparent in their stories.

Good physical health is important. Being free from injury is necessary in order to compete. It is crystal clear that none of these athletes wanted to stop participating in their games. All these sports can be defined as difficult, mentally and physically exhausting, strenuous, and extreme. You might wonder why these people are still engaging in these behaviors. What is their motivation? There are many explanations as to why the older athlete still continues competing. But there is no simple answer to the question.

Alfred Adler provides a theoretical model to better understand the underlying motivation or the 'why' factor. According to Adler, the centerpiece of his theory is the "creative self." The self is motivated to overcome and compensate for deficiencies or failings. This self accomplishes that objective by searching for particular compensating experiences and activities, by setting goals, and by developing a sense of mastery to help fulfill this uniqueness. Goal setting is a conscious activity that takes place in the present or the "here and now." By setting realistic goals the individual has to research, analyze, synthesize, think through, and plan for the future.

In order to accomplish this goal setting, the individual develops expectancies, raises levels of aspiration, improves intellectual capacity, and develops muscular and/or physical strength. As a consequence, goal setting and the accompanying behaviors result in a consistent pattern that defines the individual, resulting in a unique style. The individual's drives, interests, and behavior then take on a life of their own. Having passion in these unique activities is a necessary and a major element for life success and well-being. Also involved in this journey is a drive to make a better society by improving interpersonal relationships. Therefore, to understand the uniqueness of the person, look at his drives, thinking style, passion, and behavior patterns.

The 'why' question is best answered by: This is who I am. This is my identity. This is what I do. I do this because I can. This is how I want to be perceived by others. Can I stop competing? Why would I want to limit who I am? When you see Peyton Manning in a television commercial, what is he doing? He's laughing, playing, and throwing a football with his brother Eli. Peyton Manning's ego identity is clear; he is a professional football quarterback.

Athletes find it difficult to change who they are. Illustrations of professional athletes from my generation support that fact. Satchel Paige, the historic baseball pitcher; Gordie Howe, the hockey legend; George Blanda, the football icon—all are perfect examples of men competing in their sports beyond the age of their peers. We remember them based on what they did, what game they played. That's who they are.

Jack Sholl and Jim Steere are two examples of the self-identity model. Jack is a rower and a member of the Sons of the American Revolution. His identity is centered on being a patriot and a sculler. He volunteers and gives his time with activities pertaining to early American history. This is how others perceive him as well. The only thing that will stop him from competing in the 2011 rowing world championship is his health.

Jim Steere competed in the world Ride & Tie championship in June 2010. He passed away approximately six weeks later in August. His passion, unique style of life, goal setting, intellectual and physical development, and mission to create a better world were the epitome of Jim to the very end. On the front of the memorial brochure commemorating Jim's life was a photograph of Jim and his horse Wesob climbing up famous Cougar Rock. This photo was taken on Jim's last 100-mile Tevis Cup race when he was 80 years of age; he was the oldest person to complete the Tevis in its 56-year history. This photograph exemplifies who Jim was and how he was perceived by others—the tough competitor, the extraordinary horseman. Jim's memorial was held at a friend's ranch in Petaluma, California, and was attended by his immediate family, the San Francisco Police mounted patrol, the U.S. Park Police mounted patrol, his horse Wesob led by his son Thom, numerous Ride & Tie cohorts, many endurance friends, veterinarian buddies, and many other loyalists. The crowd was over 300 in attendance. We all loved, and continue to love Jim Steere.

Each of the young men and women in this book has accomplished so much in their athletic activities. They have developed expectancies and goals that facilitate their own style of living. They strive for perfection in order to become the very best at what they do. Their achievement, affiliation, meaning, and aggressive needs continue to be met in a healthy, admiring, inspirational environment. Each of them continues to keep the emotional components filled in a positive manner.

It is my hope that as you age, you gain new personal insights and knowledge about the many possibilities and activities open to you in your development. There are many choices to be made. Do not let old, self-defeating ideas get in the way of establishing an enriching and fulfilling life. By changing the way we think and changing our behavior, many new horizons and opportunities open up. Become the "I can" person. The sky is the limit.

Good luck.

Stay healthy, find passion, play, have fun and fulfill your own uniqueness.

Acknowledgements

I am indebted to a number of people who provided suggestions and encouragement during the development and writing of this project.

My sister Beverly Lieberman for being there as pit crew, support person, facilitator, coach, and friend. She provided great assistance at the formation stage with pertinent ideas and appropriate suggestions. Shells referred me to significant individuals like Mike Barlow who facilitated the process of getting a manuscript ready for publication.

Thank you Kate Riordan for your input and support.

A special thanks to Tony Brickel as a friend, running partner, competitor, pacer, support, and for his technical expertise. He also introduced me to the electronic world.

Many thanks to Jack Sholl, Jim Steere, Russ Kiernan, Lew Hollander, Doc Shay, Sammy Stanbro, and Beverlee Bentley for sharing with me their world.

Thank you to all my Ride & Tie, endurance, and running friends.

A heartfelt thanks to the Winter Goose staff and editors for their expertise.

I'm indebted to my wife Linda for her love, support, encouragement, and being there as my partner these past eight years. She read the entire manuscript and made valuable and honest comments that allowed me to rethink and improve it.

References

Anderson, B. (2000). *Stretching*. Shelter Publications, INC.

Berquist, L. (2009). *Second wind — The rise of the ageless athlete*. Human Kinetics.

Caldwell, P. (2006). *Molokai-Oahu, through the years*. Additions Limited.

Erikson, E.H. (1963). *Childhood & society*. WW Norton & Co.

Hall, C.S. & Lindzey, G. (1957). *Theories of personality*. John Wiley & Sons, INC.

Hollander, L. (1996). *Endurance riding*. Green Mansions.

Parsons, A., compiled by, (2010). *40 years of madness: A history of ride and tie championships*. Ride and Tie Association.

Small, G. (2006). *The longevity bible*. Hyperion.

Wilson, B.G. (1998). *Challenging the mountains: The life and times of Wendell T. Robie*. Robie Historical Foundation.

Weil, A. (2005). *Healthy aging*. Alfred A. Knopf.

Periodicals

Beck, B. (2010, March 30). Spinning blood isn't just for athletes. *The Wall Street Journal.*

Bono, Kissinger, H., & Kluger, J. (2010, May 10). 100 most influential people in the world. *Time.*

Bried, E. (2009, May). Age has nothing to do with it. *Self.*

Cloud, J. (2009, August 17). The myth about exercise. *Time.*

Dooren, J.C. (2010, March 24). New exercise goal 60 minutes a day. *The Wall Street Journal.*

Grierson, B. (2010, November 28). The incredible flying non-agrarian. *The New York Times.*

Johnson, K. (2010, January 8). Seeing old age is a never-ending adventure. *The New York Times.*

Kolata, G. (2008, January 8). Does exercise really keep us healthy. *The New York Times.*

Longman, J. (2010, November 7). After 90 vivacious years what's another marathon? *The New York Times.*

Murphy, J. (2010, December 7). A couple that runs together keeps running. *The Wall Street Journal.*

O'Connell, V. (2010, July 22). Objection older lawyers resist forced retirement. *The Wall Street Journal.*

Park, A. (2010, February 22). The science of living longer. *Time.*

Pope, T.C. (2009, October 27). The human body is built for distance. *The New York Times.*

Ruffenach, G. (2010, February 20-21). 10 best Oscar retirement films of all time. *The Wall Street Journal.*

Russo, F. (2011, January 10). Get wellness. *Time.*

Soderlund, G., & The Western States Board of Trustees. (2003, June 28). *Participant's Guide, 2003 Western States Endurance Run.*

Ride & Tie Contributors

Animal Medical Center, Large Animal Services, Drs. Doss, De Carlo, and Tarrisi, 1525 Grass Valley Hwy., Auburn, CA. 95603, 530-823-0162

Auburn Drug Company, Liz Briggs and Charlie Fink, 815 Lincoln Wy., Auburn, CA. 95603, 530-885-6524

Bright Earth Foods, Jerome Beauchamp, 916-996-8066

Cool Feed and Ranch Supply, Jody Gray, Carolynne Knisley, 2968 Highway 49, Suite M., Cool, CA. 95614, 530-87-0200

Cool Fitness, Jim and Justine Brown, 2968 State Hwy. 49, Suite D., Cool, CA. 95614, 530-823-3930

Cool Physical Therapy, James C. Kreutz, 5000 Ellinghouse Dr. #100, Cool, CA. 95614, 530-887-9598

Echo Valley Ranch, Greg Kimler, 205 Nevada St., Auburn, CA. 95603, 530-823-1482

Monsters of Massage, Ve Loyce, 455 Main St., Suite 8, Newcastle, CA. 95658, 916-663-0109

Placer County Farm Supply Cooperative, Inc., Pamela Fanini, 10120 Ophir Rd., Newcastle, CA. 95658, 916-663-3741

Scott's Automotive, Scott Hergerton, 3006 Highway 49, Suite G., Cool, CA. 95614, 530-887-1952

Sundowner of California, Christine Daniel, 505 Hilltop Dr., Auburn, CA. 85603, 530-887-9502

Sunrise Natural Foods, Teresa Gonzales, 2160 Grass Valley Hwy., Auburn, CA. 85603, 530-888-8973

The Australian Connection, Janet Pucci, 314 Dutch Ravine Ln., Newcastle, CA. 95658, 800-847-8521

Timberline Realty, Bob Sutton, Tami Sutton, and Barbara Mancia, 2968 Highway 49, Suite 80, P.O. Box 249, Cool, CA. 95614, 530-823-1088

About The Author

Frank Lieberman, PhD, is a 71-year-old psychologist, born in Detroit, Michigan, and has a professional background in teaching and clinical practice. His experience includes teaching at the elementary, junior high and secondary levels in the public schools in the Detroit area. He also was an assistant professor at Oakland Community College near Detroit. After receiving his PhD from Wayne State University in 1973, he took an assistant Professor position at Cal State San Bernardino. After leaving Cal State San Bernardino he began the practice of psychology in the San Francisco Bay area.

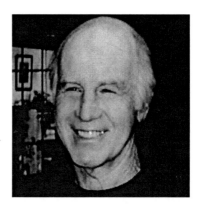

While residing in the Bay area, Dr. Lieberman began endurance riding, NATRC, and the sport of Ride & Tie. He divorced in 1999 and moved to Cool a small community in the foothills of the Sierra. This area which is near Auburn is recently classified as the endurance capital of the world. Since age 60, he has completed three one day 100 mile events called the Tevis Cup, Western states 100, and the Swanton Pacific 100 mile Ride & Tie. Since age 57 he has completed over 900 endurance miles, over 1150 running miles, and over 1850 Ride & Tie miles. He has also recently taken up the water sport of kayaking.

Frank and Linda recently married. They have five children, and seven grandchildren. He is semi-retired as a private practice psychologist. His current activities consist of play, having fun, sporting activities, writing a blog, and being healthy.

Find out more about Frank at:
http://www.ithasnothingtodowithage.blogspot.com/